THE ULTIMATE GUIDE
TO
GETTING INTO
NURSING SCHOOL

Genevieve E. Chandler, RN, PhD
Director of Second Bachelor's Program
Junior Year Writing Coordinator
School of Nursing
University of Massachusetts at Amherst
Amherst, Massachusetts

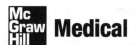 **Medical**

New York Chicago San Francisco Lisbon London Madrid Mexico City
Milan New Delhi San Juan Seoul Singapore Sydney Toronto

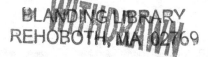

The Ultimate Guide to Getting into Nursing School

1 2 3 4 5 6 7 8 9 0   DOC/DOC   0 9 8 7

ISBN 978-0-07-147780-2
MHID 0-07-147780-2

This book was set in Plantin by International Typesetting and Composition.
The editors were Quincy McDonald and Robert Pancotti.
The production supervisor was Sherri Souffrance.
Project management was provided by International Typesetting and Composition.
The designer was Eve Siegel; the cover designer was Aimee Davis.
RR Donnelley was printer and binder.

This book is printed on acid-free paper.

Library of Congress Cataloging-in-Publication Data

Chandler, Genevieve Elizabeth.
    The ultimate guide to getting into nursing school / Genevieve E.
Chandler.
       p. ; cm.
Includes index.
ISBN-13: 978-0-07-147780-2 (pbk. : alk. paper)
ISBN-10: 0-07-147780-2
    1. Nursing schools—Admission. 2. Nursing—Vocational guidance.
I. Title.
[DNLM: 1. Schools, Nursing. 2. Education, Nursing. 3. Nursing.
WY 19 C455u 2008]
RT73.C483   2008
610.73071'1—dc22

                                                           2007022584

Contents

How to Use This Book / viii
Foreword / ix
Preface / xi
Acknowledgments / xv

[CHAPTER 1]

The Inside Story of Nursing   1
Is Nursing the Career for You?

The Inside Story / 3
A Rich, Proud History / 6
The Domains of Nursing / 12
Conclusion / 27
End-of-Chapter Exercise / 27

[CHAPTER 2]

How Do I Get There from Here?   29
Nursing as a Career / 37
Nursing Programs / 40
Conclusion / 53
End-of-Chapter Exercise / 53

[CHAPTER 3]

Self-Assessment   55
Preparing to Apply to School

Personal Inventory / 58
Be Organized / 61
Create Relationships / 73
Be Curious / 75
Be Assertive / 76
Conclusion / 77
End-of-Chapter Exercise: Letter of
    Recommendation / 78

[CHAPTER 4]

On the Right Track 81

Applications, Essays, and Interviews

The Essay / 82
Letters of Recommendation / 92
The Campus Visit / 98
The Interview / 98
Finally, What to Wear to the Interview / 101
Last, But Not Least, What if? / 102
Conclusion / 102
End-of-Chapter Exercise / 103

[CHAPTER 5]

You're In! 105

How to Be Successful Once You Get There?

What I Wish Someone Told Me . . . / 108
School and Family: Juggle or Balance? / 134
Nontraditional Students in a Traditional Program / 135
Mentoring: Good for Both Parties / 137
Conclusion / 138
End-of-Chapter Exercise: Been There, Done That / 138

[CHAPTER 6]

Moving On! 139

The Transition from Student to Nurse

The New Nurse / 140
National Counsel Licensing Exam: NCLEX / 143
Review Courses / 144
Pass, No Pass / 144
Job Search / 147
Career Services / 148
Preparing a Résumé / 148
Cover Letters / 150
Interview / 153
Dress Rehearsal / 155
A Solid Support Network / 157
A Substantial Orientation / 159

A Caring Nurse Manager / 161
A Preceptor Match / 162
Finding a Mentor / 163
Experience and Environment / 164
Conclusion / 168
End-of-Chapter Exercise / 168

[CHAPTER 7]

Going Back 171
Anticipating Graduate School

What's in it for You? / 172
Graduate School / 173
First Step / 177
What Is Graduate School Like? / 185
Doctoral Programs / 190
Conclusion / 193
End-of-Chapter Exercise / 193

[APPENDIX A]

A Sample of Assignments Required in an Introductory Nursing Course 195

[APPENDIX B]

NCLEX Preparation Resources 197

[APPENDIX C]

Web Sites with Information for Students Attending an AD (Two-Year) Degree or a BS (Four-Year) Degree 199

Index / 201

How to Use This Book

When you read the stories and answer the questions in this book, you will feel like we are having a conversation about your life. With guidance from students and nurses, you will feel like you have a mentor to guide you through important career decisions.

Stories from Current Students and Narratives from Real Nurses

Student and nursing narratives are presented throughout the book to give you a feel for what it is like to be a nurse.

- If you know what nurses do, how nurses think, and the types of roles nurses have, you will be better able to make a good career choice.
- If you have a deeper understanding of nursing, you will be able to create a better application and be more prepared for the rigors of school.

Questions to Get You Thinking

Writing out your own unique answers to critical questions will help you think through the application, the campus visit, and the interview.

Reflections to Develop Your Opinions

Thinking through the Reflective Exercises will provide you with insight into yourself and into nursing.

Chapter 1 takes you right to the bedside of the patient so you can see what it is like to give patient care.

Chapter 2 paints a picture of what it is like to be in nursing school and what to expect for coursework and classes.

Chapter 3 provides a self-assessment so that you can see how you fit into nursing and if nursing is the right fit for you.

Chapter 4 takes you step-by-step through the application process from essay to letters of recommendation.

Chapter 5 is the student perspective on "what I wish someone told me,"—advice on how to be successful in school and how to manage the stress of the nursing major.

Chapter 6 contains words of wisdom from novice nurses who have successfully made the leap from school to work.

Chapter 7 contains advice from graduate students on designing your future and how to decide to return to school.

Foreword

Simply put, I wish that I had found this book and met this author earlier in my nursing career.

The Book: Where was *this* information when *I* was considering nursing school?

Nursing school is a tornado. Unlike the usual blustery squalls of most college endeavors, it can knock you off your feet. In the course of a few short months of immersion into a nursing curriculum, you will learn a new language—yes, the field of medicine and nursing has its own grammar and its own confounding syntax. You will tackle interpersonal and intimate care-giving challenges, you will find your own threshold for nauseating experiences, and you will tell yourself, many times, "I just don't think I can do this." Eventually, however, you will see yourself doing amazing things, feeling like an imposter the whole time, but doing them nonetheless. The information in this book will prepare you for and help protect you from the storm.

If you are just launching your nursing career, or are taking a few tentative steps of inquiry, I beseech you: read this book.

The Author: I met Ginny Chandler after the tornado had hit.

After working as a nurse's aide and completing nursing prerequisite courses, I attended a fine community college nursing program in Greenfield, Massachusetts, and graduated with an Associate's Degree in Nursing. I met Ginny literally on the day that I passed the NCLEX exam to certify as a Registered Nurse. Ginny has a knack for jumping right into the middle of a student's whirlwind of thoughts and insecurities and calming the storm. Ginny kept the calm as I went on, with her encouragement, to more and more schooling.

So here it is, boiled down to a text, to calm your storm and keep you grounded while you take on the rigors of a nursing career. Nursing offers personal challenges and interpersonal connections that will lead you to an expansive, diverse, and captivating field.

Welcome.

John W. Todd, RN, MS, APRN-BC
Family Nurse Practitioner

Preface

When was the first time you thought of being a nurse? Who or what influenced your ideas about nursing? It has been said that nursing is a calling. What called you to nursing? My path to nursing began with a childhood ambition.

"I always wanted to be a nurse," my mother would say wistfully, while sitting at the kitchen table sipping her afternoon tea. "Well, why didn't you?" I'd pipe up. "My father told us that he did not come over to this country to have his daughters do that dirty work." Although each of his daughters had wanted to be a nurse, in that era when the father spoke, the children listened, so no one mentioned nursing again. That is, until my mother and her two sisters had children of their own. Each of the three sisters passed the desire to be a nurse onto their daughters. Now my cousin Davey is a surgical nurse in England, my cousin Peggy is a nurse practitioner working with abused children in Connecticut, and I became a mental health nurse and professor of nursing. The spirit of caring for those in need was handed down to the next generation.

This story from my childhood tells yourselves how I started thinking about nursing. The way in which we get to know each other is through our stories. When we meet new people, they tell us stories about where they are from, what they like to do, or the kind of music they listen to. When we see old friends, we catch up by listening to their stories. In this book, you have the chance to really get to know nursing from the stories of students and hear what it is like to be a nurse from the stories of practicing nurses. This book is designed to help you make a good career decision by examining your own thoughts about becoming a nurse and hearing from students and nurses about their experiences.

In Chapter 1, you are invited behind closed doors to see how central the role of the nurse is in providing patient care through the narratives of real nurses. Chapter 2 describes what nursing school is like from the inside view of the nursing student in an RN-to-BS program, a BS program, and a Second Bachelor's program. Chapter 3 includes a self-assessment that is designed to help you learn whether nursing is the right career for you. In Chapter 4, a step-by-step guide for developing a successful application to nursing school takes you through the process, from writing the personal essay to soliciting the appropriate letters of recommendation. We will look at postadmission interviews, how to choose between offers of acceptance, and what's the plan if you are not accepted. Chapter 5 gives you the "lowdown" on how to succeed in school and in clinical once you are accepted into a program. Given the reality of high attrition rates in nursing programs, this chapter will teach you invaluable information on how to succeed using tried-and-true study strategies and, at the same time, how to take care of yourself. You will hear words of wisdom from current nursing students, recent graduates, and faculty members on learning how to succeed in school. Chapter 6 is packed with advice from graduates on making a successful transition from a student to a nurse, including pointers on developing your resume. Chapter 7 invites you into a conversation with graduate and doctoral students about deciding whether to return to school and what you need to do to get there.

Every year, there are thousands of applicants to nursing schools. You already know that many applicants to these programs are not accepted. If you are interested in nursing, then I want you to be successful in gaining entrance into the program of your choice. This book will help you achieve your goal.

Today, with such strong competition to gain admission into nursing programs, the application process alone can make you feel overwhelmed, disorganized, and discouraged. That is where this book comes in. Let's look at the applicant picture. So who does get into nursing school? Here is the view from the admissions committee: There are applicants who apply to nursing programs with high GPAs and good SAT scores and some who apply who are on the lower end. However, *the majority of accepted applicants, wait-listed applicants, and those who are not admitted look remarkably similar.* What I mean is that many applicants have similar qualifications. Oh, some applicants are on the high end for GPAs and some on the low end, but the majority of applicants would do well in nursing school and would make fine nurses. So how do you stand out from the competition? How do you move into the "Accept" category? Developing an understanding of what it is like to be a nurse, taking the application process seriously, getting into school, and doing well can be accomplished at once because applying to school, succeeding in school, and performing as a practicing nurse all require similar skills. This book will help you identify and hone those necessary skills. The bottom line is that our patients need you, so let's get going!

With help from the interactive features contained in this book, we will have a conversation about your future. The information in these pages will empower you to be in the best possible position to be accepted into the nursing program of your choice. By engaging in this conversation, you will come to understand why you want to pursue nursing and you will be prepared to write a sterling application that is unique, thoughtful, and focused. This interactive text features provocative questions and specifically designed opportunities for you to respond with your thoughts and ideas to clarify your own opinion and formulate your own unique position. The stories in this book are real, the advice is from the inside, and the conversation is created for you.

Let's start right now by reflecting back on other projects you have successfully accomplished. This is where we have a conversation. Now you talk to me. Ready? Your turn.

Reflective Thinking

Applying to nursing school is taking on a new project. Think back at a time when you wanted to do something new, like play on the softball team, perform in a play, or get a good grade on a test. Identify one new project you have already taken on in your life.

What is the project you are thinking of?

Now, list four things that you did to prepare yourself for that project:

1.

2.

3.

4.

Whom did you go to for help in getting ready to try out?

Who provided you with encouragement to succeed?

Preparing to take on something new takes time. You need to learn what the new project requires, whether it is trying out for a team, being chosen for a play, or applying to nursing school. To succeed in any new project takes practice. Practice means organizing your life so that you have time to get ready. The key words here are *organizing* and *time*. Last minute, the night before, or even the week before will not work for sports, theater, or school. Next, you will obtain critical information by talking with people who have done this before and by learning what you need to do to be successful. It is essential to identify those persons who have supported you and those who have encouraged you to keep going. You will need mentors and a support network for this project too. The good news is that you have been success-ful at other projects by being prepared, having support, and learning from those who went before you. The guidance offered in the Ultimate Guide to Getting into Nursing School will prepare you to be successful in this proj-ect of deciding and pursuing a career in nursing.

Acknowledgments

I would like to express my sincere appreciation to all of the students who offered their precious words for publication. Traditional undergraduates, returning RNs, and second bachelor's, master's, and doctoral students courageously provided the intimate descriptions of the nurse–patient relationship and a window into the life of a student. The clinical narratives submitted by undergraduate students were the product of the "Writing in Ethics" class, in which students had the opportunity to write from their heart, receive peer editing, and rewrite their drafts with coaching from the instructor. The results offer a rare opportunity for readers to experience the hidden details of care and the private voice of the nurse to aid in this important career decision. A sincere "thank you" to all who have submitted their work to be considered for *The Ultimate Guide to Getting into Nursing School.*

CHAPTER 1

The Inside Story of Nursing

Is Nursing the Career for You?

So you want to be a nurse? Great idea! The first step is to get into nursing school. Let's start the school application process by taking a close look at what it is like to be a nurse, how nurses think, and what they actually do. Knowing the inside story of nursing will help you to create a stronger application to nursing school.

In this chapter, you will have the opportunity to shadow a nurse in different areas of practice. Practicing nurses and student nurses will take us behind closed doors to see what it is like to actually care for patients, to collaborate with physicians, and to manage a complex case. Nurses have a rich, proud history of providing patient care, coordinating health care teams, and developing local, national, and global health policy. Before we get to the future, though, let's start by finding out what nursing is all about so you can make sure the role of a nurse fits with your career goals.

Meet Emi, a new student nurse, who takes us into the pediatric unit:

Annie, a 6-week-old infant, was admitted from the ER with multiple fractures of the clavicle, skull, and ribs, and retinal hemorrhaging from a diagnosis of shaken baby syndrome. Shaken baby syndrome often occurs when a parent or caretaker becomes so frustrated with their baby's crying that they pick the baby up and shake the infant so hard that the baby's retinas detach, which causes permanent blindness. When I walked into her room, I found a tiny baby lying in the middle of a large metal crib. Her thick black hair was flattened against her head with a pink bow on top. At first, I was overwhelmed by

Annie's cuteness and the sadness of her story, which suddenly became real when I saw how small and delicate she was. I began to wonder what I could possibly do for this baby and I was afraid of breaking her further. As a nurse, what could I do to help her heal? I knew what she needed was to repair her bones and injuries, which would require good nutrition, rest, and pain management. Annie also had suffered a complete breakdown of trust when a parent injured her so severely. I knew my role was not only to help her heal the physical wounds that this abuse had left but to address the overwhelming emotional and developmental toll as well. I spent much of the shift holding her in my arms, providing closeness. My pediatric instructor often reminded our class that sick and injured children not only need interventions in the form of treatment for their ailments but also the regular, supportive care children need to grow. I looked for signs of pain so she could get the correct pain medication, I looked for intracranial pressure by assessing the pitch of her cry, the alignment of her eyes, the change in blood pressure. While feeding Annie, I assessed her neurological status, knowing a poor suck and lack of tracking movements of her eyes were indications of her conditions.

Emi reflects, "My care of Annie is a good example of the work of nursing, often invisible to the untrained eye. From the hallway it simply appeared I was a young woman holding a baby but so much more was really happening."

Emi, as a novice student, already understands what is meant when nurses are described as "knowledge workers." A knowledge worker is someone who carries much of what they are doing in their head. We don't always see what is going on when we see a nurse with a patient. For example, in this case, Emi looks as if she is just tending to a tiny baby, but she is really conducting a thorough head-to-toe assessment for neurological changes while assessing baby Annie for pain. Emi is attending to Annie's comfort, giving the appropriate medications and maintaining the important human connection a baby needs. In many of the narratives in this book, it will appear that the nurse is doing something simple, but in reality, the thought processes are very complex. The work of a nurse can be hard to see from the outside. For example, when a nurse walks into a room to greet a new patient, while he is asking about the patient's day, he is noticing the patient's breathing. Is Mrs. Smith's breathing labored or normal? When he is asking about the patient's day, he is assessing her mental status. Is she confused? Is she aware of where she is and why she is here? The nurse may be making casual conversation about the weather while he is examining the patient's IV to see if the solution is flowing properly. As he gently holds the patient's hand, he is making sure the IV insertion site is not swollen. There is a lot going on when the nurse is asking the patient, "How are you today?" By reading the following stories, you will gain an understanding of what nursing is all about so that when you apply to school you will feel confident that you've made the right career decision. Your confidence in your decision is a step toward creating a successful school application.

THE INSIDE STORY

The majority of prenursing students envision themselves cuddling a new baby, wiping the brow of a fevered young man, or holding the hand of an elderly widow. Providing comfort is an important part of the nurse's role, but there is so much more. The nurse is the critical link between the patient, the family, and the rest of the health care team. The nurse teaches the patient about the illness, the nurse communicates the patient's and family's concerns to the physician, the nurse calls in the social worker, consults with the chaplain, and connects the patient to hospital and community resources. Oh, I know, you are saying what 80 percent of the first year nursing students say, "I want to take care of kids or work in labor and delivery," and they picture healthy kids and perfect babies. Sometimes that happens, but often the scene is more complex. The other day, my students came back from their first clinical day on the maternity unit reporting, "Oh, it is interesting but the three new moms were 14 and 15 years old, it would be hard for me to work with such young mothers." Here Laurie, a nurse expert, invites us into her practice as a labor and delivery nurse:

Angela and Peter arrived on our unit from their doctors' office. They were serious, shaken, and holding back tears. What was I to say to a family that had just heard such devastating news? They had just learned that their unborn baby would not survive the day. A diagnosis of Trisomy 18 was recited to them. This devastating genetic trick had happened to their child. Unlike Trisomy 21, commonly known as Down syndrome, the defect that their baby will be born with is a defect with a cardiac abnormality that is incompatible with life. I simply said, "I'm sorry," and held both of their hands for a moment, the first of many intimate times to come.

Nurses are there with patients during birth, life, and death. In this case, Laurie and her patients, the young couple and their unborn baby, experience birth, life, and death all within a few hours. Before Angela and Peter came to the nurse, the physician pronounced the diagnosis of Trisomy 18. Laurie listened carefully to their concerns, anticipated what would be needed and developed a plan with the parents to address their needs:

At a time like this, the nurse needs to be comfortable attending to physical and emotional concerns. This family needs vital signs, monitoring contractions, IV, and blood work all done between sobs. Peter, the husband, kept busy making hushed phone calls to family and friends. He asked aloud, "Who would tell the children? Would they come to the hospital?" Having their children close is what they would always do in times of distress. My mind kept asking, "Why not now? What would people think? Having children here especially at a time like this? Am I out of line as a nurse?" Funeral, burial, what awful things to think about! Never mind having to ask a grieving family these questions, but it's my job to ask. Baby death brings such a torrent of the unimaginable. There are avenues to choose and no road map to help navigate. I would have to create the map and guide this family through the unknown territory. Would they see their baby? Would they hold her after her delivery? Each family directs the ballet of emotional twirls that balance the tears with the tasks. Our Bereavement Program helps me to formulate a plan to complete each area of need while my own emotions are heightened.

Laurie reflected, "At times like this, I know I'm in the right profession, I'm a nurse and I'm proud that I am willing and able to guide and support this family. Caring for this family made me a better human. They gave me permission to help other families by testing the scary waters of death. I am no longer afraid of being weird by offering rituals that force us to be present. I can offer what worked for another family and support them through their loss, the loss of a child, the ultimate loss".

As a nurse, you can work with the newborn babies, the frail, the elderly, and everyone in between. You can work in the intensive care unit with critically ill patients and their families, or as a visiting nurse going out to patient's homes, or in a middle school, attending to adolescents as a school nurse. There are challenges in every situation. Take the school nurse; that is a familiar role. We've all been to school. We think we know what the school nurse does: we read the eye chart back to the nurse, hold up our finger if we hear a beep in our ear, and head for the nurse's office when we scrap our knee. Yup, that is part of the job, but there is much more. Virginia writes about her day as a school nurse:

Melissa, a 14-year-old female, came into the school nurse office early one October morning. "Mrs. Hyde, my mom asked me to have you take a look at my rash," she stated as she exposed her arm to me. Melissa added, "The doctor looked at it last week and said he thought it might be an allergy to my cat," she commented. "I don't see anything here on your arm Melissa, tell me more about it," I queried.

My mind was clicking fast; I definitely didn't like the "sweaty at night" statement. Melissa attributed this to the fact that her cat slept on her chest and he was making her hot at night. As I further investigated her "cold" symptoms I took her temperature. I began my mental assessment. This is a 14-year-old female with a history of rash for two weeks, chest cold for several months, night sweats, and maybe a low-grade temperature. What childhood illnesses often present themselves with night sweats? My mind races and I come up with three possibilities. "Melissa, do you cough often?" I inquire. "Yes, I do," she replies. "And when you do cough, does anything come up; do you produce any phlegm?" She denies a productive cough, informing me that it is more of a dry cough. I know what is wrong; I can't believe no one has picked this up! Then I begin to question myself. "Please God, don't let this be what I think it is," I said to myself.

In this case, Virginia is conducting a nursing assessment while drawing on her vast clinical knowledge and developing a possible diagnosis of Melissa's condition.

Melissa's temperature was 99.8. I was so happy she had a temperature. State law requires us to send all students home with a temperature of 99 or above. If I sent her home, someone besides me could investigate my suspicions. I really wanted to refer her back to her physician right away. With a temperature, I not only was able to send her home, but I was required to notify her mother immediately.

Unfortunately, my suspicions were correct. Melissa was admitted to the hospital with a diagnosis of Hodgkin's disease. Melissa didn't return to school that year. I visited the hospital on and off through the course of her illness. Melissa died 18 months after the day she came to see me. Somehow, she knew something was seriously wrong with her. At 14 years old, Melissa had the fortitude to continue to seek medical advice for symptoms that were vague and nondescript, and I knew, when a variety of vague symptoms occur, to very carefully and systematically ask questions and conduct a thorough follow-through. The results of Melissa's case only reinforced the responsibility I have for "my" children. Melissa will remain forever in my mind and I will always have place for her in my heart.

Nurses play a critical role from schools to intensive care units. Can you picture yourself in the neonatal intensive care unit (NICU) where baby Annie was, or as a school nurse seeing 65 cases a day? What nursing role fits you?

Each Reflection in this book is designed to help you think through your idea of being a nurse. For each Reflection, actually write out your answer. Writing your words on the page takes your thoughts out of your head and lets you examine your thoughts from a distance, on the page, so that you can play with your ideas and maybe come up with new ways of thinking.

Reflection 1: Where Do You See Yourself as a Nurse?

1. Have you envisioned being a certain type of nurse?

2. Where do you see yourself practicing in 5 years?

3. Take a moment to describe your career dream, being as specific as possible.

4. Every area of nursing has a professional organization. Once you have identified your interest, visit the following web site to learn more about your preferred area of nursing: http://www.nurse.org/orgs.

A RICH, PROUD HISTORY

In the popular media, nurses are depicted trailing after physicians, jotting down every request while answering the call light for rooms filled with grateful patients. Or the nurse is seen barking orders and demanding that patients be obedient, just as Nurse Ratched did in *One Flew Over The*

Cuckoo's Nest. Historically, nurses typically are pictured as docile in spirit and silent in voice. In fact, back in the 1800s, a nurse was required to be single, and unattractive (honestly, so they would not distract patients). When training to be a nurse, the students were required to live in a dorm at the end of the hall of the hospital unit so that the student was available to meet every patient's and doctor's need. Back then, hospitals were staffed by student nurses. When the nurse graduated from school, she no longer worked in a hospital but was hired out for private duty or worked out in the community in the neighborhood clinic. The image of silent, subservient nurse reflects the Victorian role of women. In reality, while maintaining the role of a proper Victorian woman, nurses could be brilliant statisticians and savvy politicians, such as Florence Nightingale, the founder of modern nursing. Florence Nightingale went into nursing in her early 20s, rebelling against her parents' wishes for her to find a husband and settle down. Instead, Ms Nightingale chose to start a career, developing nursing into a profession. Read her compelling story on this web site, http://www.spartacus.schoolnet.co.uk.

In the 1870's, nurses led by Margaret Sanger lobbied for much needed birth control for the poor and destitute. Check out http://womenshistory. about.com/library/bio/blbio_margaret_sanger.htm. At the beginning of the 20th century, Lillian Wald was one of the nurses who pioneered neighborhood health programs that addressed the immigrants devastating needs of the community. Read more at http://www.jwa.org/exhibits/wov/wald/.

These great women were responding to the needs of their patients not only at the bedside with individuals but also out in the community with families and across the globe in war-torn nations. From her office in London, Ms Nightingale developed a national plan to attend to wounded soldiers in the Crimean War, 100 years before "globalization" was even a concept!

From the beginnings of professional nursing to the present day, responding to the needs of the patient has been central to the role of the nurse. As Virginia Henderson, a nursing leader, so elegantly stated, "A nurse does for the patient what the patient would do for themselves if they had the strength, knowledge and wherewithal."

The unique function of the nurse is to assist the individual, sick or well, in the performance of those activities contributing to health or its recovery (or to peaceful death) that he would perform unaided if he had the necessary strength, will or knowledge. And to do this in such a way as to help him gain independence as rapidly as possible (Henderson, 1966, p. 15).

Ellyn, an expert rehabilitation nurse, demonstrates how she assisted her patient in the activities that would lead to recovery and independence:

Pictures on Paulo's bedside table told the story of a confident and strong 22-year-old male with smooth dark skin, a lean muscular body, and dark hair that hung in loose curls around his smiling tanned face. The half dozen or so colorfully framed snapshots revealed an active thrill-seeking Paulo who enjoyed water sports and outdoor activities. All the pictures I saw were a stark contrast to the frail, uncoordinated, wounded body that lay in the bed before me.

I learned from reading his hospital chart that Paulo was in this country illegally when he rolled his Nissan pickup truck off a back country road after a night of heavy drinking and snorting drugs at a late night party. After his rescue by local first responders, he spent two months in a coma in the intensive care unit. Although Paulo was no longer in a coma, no longer intubated, and no longer being tube-fed when he arrived as an inpatient on the rehabilitation unit, he still had a lot of healing to do if he was ever going to regain the level of functioning and independence he enjoyed before his accident. It was my job to help Paulo adjust to his situation by listening to him while he processed what he had just come through, encouraging him through the sometimes painful therapies that lay ahead, and to teach him how to care for himself so he could be as independent as possible. I knew those things were in our future, but for now I tended to his immediate needs.

I checked the Foley catheter tube that extended from his body to the collection bag hanging below the bedside to be sure it was patent. I assessed the urine flowing into it for color, clarity, and amount. I closely observed the white gauze dressings covering the open wounds over several parts of his body to see if there was any drainage coming from them and if there were any signs or symptoms of infection. There was a G-tube protruding from Paulo's abdomen that was no longer being used to sustain his life but would remain intact until there was sufficient evidence of weight gain to indicate he was consuming enough calories by mouth to keep him healthy. I noted its insertion site was clean, dry, and without any redness, all signs the tube was not recently inserted. Paulo was barely aware of the tubes and dressings covering his thin weak body as I carefully checked each one during my assessment.

As Paulo's memories of the accident gradually penetrated back into his conscious, his agitation decreased and his impulsiveness diminished. He shared with me some of his memories of what happened as I listened quietly and without judgment.

For Ellyn and Paulo, this is just the first hour of a 12-hour shift. You can hear what is going through Ellyn's mind as she is assessing Paulo, considering his past, tending to his present state, and anticipating his future.

So let's apply the definition of nursing to back to our case with Paulo. If Paulo could take care of himself while he was recovering from a coma, he would not need a nurse. He would do what the nurse was doing for him: keep up his nutrition, change his dressings, and relearn to walk and try to understand how to piece the life back together. But that is not possible for a patient this ill, so that is where the nurse comes in: *developing a plan to assist the patient to do what is needed to become healthy again.*

Okay, now we are getting serious here about what you will be doing as a nurse, so listen carefully . . .

The brief definition of nursing includes: "nurses diagnose and treat how people respond to their illness." Let's think about what this definition means. The definition identifies that the nurse's focus is the *response to illness, not just the illness itself.* For Paulo, his illness is a head injury, broken bones, and a destroyed self-image. His *response* to his head injury, broken bones, and a destroyed self-image is what Ellyn attended to. Let me explain. His head injury was treated in the ER when he first entered the hospital. You can picture him being rushed in the ambulance from the grizzly scene of the accident, rolled on a stretcher into the ER, right? After his critical injuries are taken care of that night in the ER, for the next three months Ellyn addressed how Paulo responded to his brain injury. In the OR, shortly after his admission, his broken bones were repaired. For the following three months, Ellyn changed the dressings, taught Paulo about managing his pain, coached him in learning about his medications, and encouraged him to participate in physical therapy so that his bones would heal. In the moments following his accident, it was obvious his self-image would be totally altered. For three months, Ellyn provided a listening ear and the personal counseling to help him process what his new identity would be like.

The first three weeks of Paulo's rehabilitation program were filled with progress. I cheered as he made great gains in mobility, stability, independence, and cognition. Nobody knew how far he would eventually progress, but it was soon clear to everyone but Paulo that he would never be able to go back to his previous job as a professional residential tree climber. I knew from our many revealing conversations that Paulo identified strongly with his occupation. It's what brought him to this country and it's what provided him with the professional respect and financial means to remain here. Paulo's job as a tree climber utilized his now-lost skills of balance, coordination, and quick thinking while also providing him with the excitement of an adrenaline high. The adrenaline rushes that excited Paulo when he was tree climbing were probably the same adrenaline rushes he was pursuing the night he made the drug and alcohol influenced choice to speed recklessly down a dark curvy road, flipping his truck and landing upside down next to a tree where his injured body laid barely alive and forever changed both physically and mentally. Now Paulo's life focused on replacing adrenaline rushes with a daily struggle to regain his independence. I educated him on the use of pain medications before therapy instead of waiting until after his therapy. I patiently explained to him that taking medication before he had any pain would allow him to work longer and harder during his therapy sessions, making his efforts more effective. I provided Paulo with information on outpatient services, scheduled his follow-up appointments with therapists, and gave him a list of where to locate drug and alcohol counseling resources in the community. As I was selectively choosing my final words of farewell, it occurred to me that what seemed to be a comprehensive discharge plan was really only a collection of well-intentioned suggestions. It was ultimately Paulo's decision what path his continued rehabilitation was going to take.

As I watched Paulo clumsily pack his belongings and prepare to leave the hospital, I seized one final opportunity for a heartfelt talk with him about his life and his future. I pulled up a nearby chair and sat down slowly as I asked Paulo to take a break from packing and join me. I spoke softly and maternally about his fragile healing brain and its need for gentle caring to support his continued progress. A healthy lifestyle for Paulo meant living a completely different lifestyle than what he lived before his accident. It meant no more drinking and drugs, no more late nights and irregular schedules, and no more tree climbing.

As expected, Paulo continued to reject the idea of being a grounds man even as he unsteadily resumed packing his belongings to leave the hospital. "I am a tree climber," was the mantra Paulo chanted to me whenever I brought up the subject. I convinced myself that perhaps he just needed some time to consider his options before accepting the fact that he may never again experience the thrill of a climb.

Two months after Paulo left the hospital, I saw him again at a local department store. As he walked toward me from the far end of the aisle, the nurse in me silently assessed his pace and balance. I watched him walk determinedly with a gait that barely told the story of a long difficult struggle back to independence. He smiled as he reached his hand out to me and said, "Hello, it is me." As I stood there with Paulo in front of me talking about his life since leaving the hospital, I was also looking to see if he had gained or lost any weight. I listened carefully to his words to determine if his speech had continued to improve. I watched his hands and fingers closely as I searched for evidence of the fine motor skills necessary to cook, clean, and dress himself. With a half-smile on his face and the familiar warm sparkle in his eyes, Paulo said, "Ellyn, I am now a grounds man. It's a lucky climber that has me under him. Thank you for helping me to see this." I understood immediately the significance of what Paulo was saying. He turned the task of redefining his self-identity into a successful joust against adversity.

Notice that, even meeting her former patient out in the community, Ellyn can't help but be a nurse, assessing Paulo's physical condition, language ability, and fine motor skills. You can begin to see why in any nursing program a course in anatomy, a course in nutrition, and a course in care for the acutely injured is required. Nursing is a complex, multilayered process. A rehabilitation nurse has the opportunity to spend more time with a patient during their healing process. Each individual has their own personal response to an illness and their own personal response to the treatment of the illness. The nurse needs to know about the illness, the treatment, and also needs to learn about their patient's individual response to their illness and their individual response to their treatment. Ed, a student nurse, describes his approach to providing care that is designed to meet the individual patient's needs:

Paul had a complete laryngectomy, which is removal of his voice box. He was a three-pack-a-day smoker who developed lung cancer. When I met him, he was lying in bed with a central line (a catheter inserted through the chest into the heart for fluids and medicines), a feeding tube, and a tracheotomy, with both his hands and feet restrained due to his alcohol withdrawal. My immediate impression was one of pity when I looked down and realized he couldn't even scratch his nose if he wanted to. From the surgery, his neck was red, bruised, and grotesquely swollen. I wondered if he would live to see the next sunrise.

The next morning, to my genuine surprise, Paul was alert and oriented but very aggravated. He was covered in his own urine and he was drooling from the left side of his mouth. His room was a disaster, with gauze in his bed, dried blood on the floor, secretions all over his chest, and used equipment strewn on his night table. I pulled the curtain closed separating his bed from his roommate and went to work.

The first day we were both very frustrated. Due to airway changes from surgery his verbal communication was lost. I was frustrated because I could not understand his hand gestures. He was frustrated because I could not understand his attempts to communicate. Somewhere along the way, it occurred to one of us that writing would be the most effective way of communicating. I obtained a white board and some markers and suddenly his demands for care became more manageable.

At the end of the day, Ed reflected, "As the shift progressed, I realized I looked forward to talking to Paul. As our relationship developed, he would allow me to guess what his hands were saying before he wrote because I believe the white board gave us both confidence to fall back on. Paul became one of those patients I will never forget."

Ed adjusted his care so that Paul could communicate. Ed addressed both the science and art of illness. The science would be: What is causing Paul's response to surgery? What symptoms should the patient expect to experience? How is lung cancer usually treated? How is lung cancer prevented? In this case, Ed used his knowledge of the science of nursing to take care of the patient's chest tubes, his central line, and his feeding tube. It is essential that Ed has the knowledge of the body, the disease, and the treatments. In addition, Ed employed the art of nursing by developing an understanding of how his patient responded to his illness, how Paul managed his symptoms, and how he handled the surgery. The role of the nurse is to attend to the patient's unique physical, emotional, and social responses.

In the following section, the responsibilities of the nurse are identified. Learning about different aspects of the nurse's role will broaden your own view of the nursing profession.

THE DOMAINS OF NURSING

To understand more fully what a nurse knows and what a nurse does, the nurse-scientist Patricia Benner studied the role of the nurse by observing nurses in practice and interviewing nurses about their experience. Dr. Benner concluded that the nurse has at least seven different roles.

The seven nursing roles are:

1. Helping role
2. Teaching-coaching function

3. Diagnostic and monitoring function

4. Effective management of rapidly changing conditions

5. Administering and monitoring therapeutic interventions

6. Monitoring and insuring quality health practices

7. Organizational functions

Helping Role

There are five aspects of the helping role of the nurse:

1. Provide relief from pain.

2. Provide comfort, offer emotional support.

3. Be present for the patient.

4. Support the patient in participating in their own care.

5. Interpret information and assist the patient in developing an understanding of their illness, just like the patient would do for themselves, if they were well enough.

Managing pain is a key component of the nursing role. The body cannot heal if it is reacting to pain. The nurse is the professional who spends the most time with the patient, and who has the opportunity to assess the patient's response to pain. With nursing education and clinical experience, the nurse learns to assess the patient's response to the pain of illness and the pain of intervention. The nurse develops a pain management plan that preserves the patient's dignity and provides the comfort needed to heal. Rick, a new student nurse, became the patient's advocate to assist in managing his pain:

My first exposure to Chester was in report when he was referred to as "the patient from hell." I walked through his door to greet an extremely anxious and fearful man. When I asked about his pain, he noted his pain was 10 on a 10-point scale. I discussed this with my preceptor who remarked, "He has been a constant complainer." I found myself becoming angry with such an insensitive comment. I decided to advocate for Chester by collecting the data from the hospital's philosophy on effective pain management and its impact on the well-being of the patient. After what seemed like an eternity, we agreed to assess Chester together. We found Chester increasingly anxious due to his pain level, but I could feel a change in attitude from my preceptor. He apologized for doubting me and seeming so insensitive. We immediately came up with a plan incorporating a medication change and alternative pain relief methods of visualization and breathing techniques. Thirty minutes later, I visited Chester and it was like I was talking to a different patient. He was level-headed and in the mood to share stories about his life.

Rick knew the role of the nurse is to *manage pain and advocate* for the patient. Through effective pain management the patient can *actively partici-pate in their own care*, even pediatric patients. Student nurse Kim reports:

Mia was a 7-year-old patient at Shriner's for a cleft palate repair. She had already had six surgeries in her short life. Her two medical files were both three inches thick. She was two days post-op and wanted to go home, though she still had considerable swelling in her mouth and lips and her right hip was sore at the point where the bone was removed to repair the palette. She was afraid to move, but to be discharged the most important thing was for Mia to get out of bed. When I mentioned getting up, tears welled up in her eyes; she was scared of the pain. I hoped to gain enough of her trust so by the end of the day she would let me help her get out of bed. We spent time coloring, drawing, and sculpting with Play-Doh. I talked with her about her dog and best friend. Later, I spoke to the nurse about administering pain medication before we got her out of bed. I told Mia both her mother and I would help her and we would go very slowly. I could see how scared she was but she was determined. She managed to walk a few steps. I was really proud of her. Later, I went in to say goodbye, Mia very shyly pulled out a drawing and handed it to me. It was a picture of Mia and me (in my school uniform) holding hands, and she had written, "Thank you for helping me Kim, Love Mia."

Kim reports, "I still have that drawing hanging on my fridge at home."

From adults experiencing pain to children who are suffering, the nurse creates a treatment plan that fits with the particular patient.

In the helping role, the nurse *provides comfort* through communication and touch. This student, Brianna, was new on the job, but with her prepa-ration from her classes and the sensitivity she brought to the job, she knew what to do:

Mrs. M. has been living in this hospital room for three weeks. She reports no physical pain. She has no difficulty with mobility or taking care of herself yet, due to arterial insufficiency her wound on her right ankle was not healing. This leads to osteomyelitis, for which she receives aggressive intravenous antibiotic treatment. She has been waiting for three weeks to have surgery to bypass an obstruction in her right femoral artery with an artificial vessel graft. She cannot go home because insurance won't sufficiently cover the cost of the antibiotic treatment if she leaves the hospital. She is staring at her legs in disgust.

"These things (her legs) are just terrible, aren't they? I guess they are dying."

The physician stops in and after a two second search for a pedal (ankle) pulse he announces, "There is no circulation in this foot, you sure need that surgery, my dear." He gives her a quick grin and leaves the room as he is jotting on his clip board. Mrs. M. slowly removes her glasses and compulsively cleans the lenses with a tissue. She bows her head and slowly says, "Never get old. Never get old."

No one has told Mrs. M. that she will not be leaving this room. "I'd like to check your pulses using a Doppler," I announce. I explain that with the Doppler you can hear pulses that sometimes are not strong enough to be felt.

"I don't mind. Do whatever you need to do."

I apply a small amount of gel on the top of her foot and move the instrument gently over the surface of her peeling skin. The machine crackles with static, then regularizes into a steady beat, beat, beat.

"What is that? Do you hear that?"

Her eyes widen and dart back and forth. Her forehead wrinkles with concern. Now she thinks her ears are failing her.

"That is your pulse in your foot."

"In my foot?"

It is the first time I have heard her indicate that her lower limbs are a part of herself.

Beat, beat, beat.

I turn the volume all the way up.

We sit back and let her pedal pulse sing in our ears.

Comfort for Mrs. M was provided by listening to her concerns, becoming aware of her sense of loss, and responding to what she needed. Often, what a patient needs is to have an interested, caring individual be with them to witness their experience. The nurse learns that being fully present for the patient initiates the healing relationship. Though on TV nurses are seen running around yelling orders, often the most healing approach can be accomplished by standing still and being quiet with the patient, *being fully present* in the moment. Being fully present means not thinking what you should have done before you walked into the room or what you could be doing when you leave the room but, rather, taking a deep breath and focusing on this patient right here, right now. This full attention can facilitate a healing interaction, just as a new student nurse, Leanne, did:

When I first met Mrs. G., it was only my second time with a patient in my role as a student nurse. As I approached the bedside, I had the same feelings of anxiety, fear, and inadequacy that took hold on my first day of clinical, that made my hands clammy and my heart race. These feelings rushed through my head, pushing out all the knowledge I had learned over the past three years. Somehow in the midst of wondering what to say, how to say it, and what to do first, I managed to utter something about the flowers on her windowsill. The next thing I knew, I found myself standing at the patient's bedside holding up a picture frame, talking to her, not about her pain, symptoms, vital signs, or bowel movements, but about her son, daughter, and her two grandsons.

Once I established rapport with Mrs. G, it was time to start the physical nursing care. I noticed in that short time since we first met something had changed; I no longer felt like an intruder. This occurred to me when it came time to help her bathe because I didn't feel like an awkward stranger anymore. I was now an assistant, a friend, a nurse. So we helped each other. "I can wash what I can while you change my linens and make my bed, then you can help me with the rest," she said to me. After battling three different kinds of cancer, being in the hospital was nothing new to her. Mrs. G taught me a lot that day and I was very grateful to her.

The nurse and patient work in collaboration to promote health and healing.

The nurse can become a *liaison for the family*, from simple gestures to complex communication. In this situation, Meghan, a new nursing student, served the patient and his family:

"Mr. P. wants a shave," my clinical instructor told me. "Okay," I said on my exhale. Only then did I realize I had been holding my breath, nervous about my first patient. "You'll be fine," she said. Mr. P. is an Italian man who used to be fluent in English, but after a series of strokes and heart attacks, converses in Italian only. I can't recall his face in detail—just the gray stubble that covered his cheeks, chin, and upper lip, and his eyes: bluish gray and lucid. His sister-in-law, an attractive dark-haired woman in her 50s, sat at his bedside.

I filled the basin with warm water and moistened his face with a cloth. I applied the shaving cream to his face haphazardly, removed the razor's cover, and turned toward Mr. P., tool in hand. I touched the razor to his face and began to shave downward, gently, on his left cheek, then moved to the right one. The disposable razor grated across his skin—scrape, scrape.

Mr. P. aided my endeavor by contorting his face, stretching out the skin between his nose and upper lip, then in the opposite direction to smooth out his chin. During this process, as I gingerly steadied his head with one hand, we met eyes and I smiled. Mr. P. smiled at me. In the corner of my eye, I could see his sister-in-law smile to herself. Our moment of connection had a witness. Her private recognition moved me.

I finished the shave, leaving some stubble here and there. I asked Mr. P.'s sister-in-law how to say handsome in Italian. "Bello," she told me. "Bello," I said to Mr. P. victoriously. He nodded respectfully. Bello, indeed.

Megan reflects, "shaving, a simple task, a menial task. A shave has little to do with medicine. But when you are a man who once ruled his house, a man who could silence his children with a glance, who shaved his own face nearly every day of his adult life, a clean-shaven face is a symbol of manhood, of dignity, and of honor." Through Megan's nursing care, she provided the gift of dignity to her patient.

Teaching patients and their families is a central nursing role. The nurse teaches and coaches in almost every patient contact.

Teaching-Coaching Function

The nurse teaches the patients about their illness, about their therapy, about their medication, and about their journey to health or a peaceful death. The patient learns about breast-feeding, how to change their own dressings, what to expect from medication, and how to recognize side effects of medication from the nurse. Teaching and learning is a complex process when an individual is well; when ill many dimensions are added. The process for teaching patients has five components:

1. Capturing the patient's readiness to learn
2. Assisting the patient to integrate their illness and recovery into their lives
3. Eliciting the patient's understanding of illness
4. Providing an interpretation of the patient's condition and a rationale for procedures
5. Making difficult aspects of illness approachable and understandable. (Benner, 1984)

Kelly talks about capturing a teachable moment:

Eighteen-year-old Dan was completing a carpentry job when the electric saw fell adjacent to his leg. Dan instinctively shoved the saw, forfeiting two right-hand fingers to the razor sharp tool. When I walked into Dan's room, he was aimlessly glancing towards the window, adorned in a hospital gown with a Boston Red Sox hat pulled down so far that it completely shaded his eyes. I inspected the area around the dressing monitoring for redness, purulent drainage, warmth, and other signs of infection. Dan quietly responded to my questions, "No" he did not feel nauseated, "yes" his pain had decreased. I explained to Dan that, with the help of my instructor, I would be changing his dressing. I suggested to Dan that we needed to teach him the proper cleaning and dressing change technique. It was then I noticed, in Dan's facial expression, anxiety and fear. "Have you seen your hand since surgery, Dan?" I inquired gently. "No, the nurse changed it last night but I couldn't look yet," Dan replied. "I can imagine that would be difficult for you," I said as I took a seat beside his bed. Dan's eyes drifted from the window onto my face as he spoke "It really is and I feel stupid because they are fingers, it is not like a leg or anything." I assured Dan that his body had been altered and what he felt was not stupid. Dan continued to disclose that he had planned on becoming a police officer, a future that had been dashed within moments. And what about when people met him for the first time, and they noticed he only had two fingers on his right hand. How would these people view him? He also admitted he was apprehensive that he would no longer be capable of what were once everyday activities, such as eating and dressing. I was honest with Dan, confirming that his life would change in some respects. Yet, I assured him he would receive help to overcome these challenges. In the end of our conversation, Dan even determined he may consider a career as a lawyer or a judge.

Following our talk, Dan was capable of looking at his hand. As I unraveled the bandage, Dan inspected the surgical site. As I patiently watched Dan observe his hand, he took a deep breath and said, "Yep, I am ready. I can do this now."

Dan was discharged later that evening with his family at his side and his baseball cap resting high on his head, his eyes clearly visible to the outside world.

Kelly addressed all five of the teaching components: readiness to learn, assisting Dan to integrate his injury into his life, listening to Dan's story, explaining the treatment, and making the injury approachable. Nurses play such a critical role in their patient's recovery process. Creating an emotional space to heal is rewarding, but in today's world it is challenging to find the time. Hospitalized patients are very ill and only in the hospital for a limited time, and the nurse is very busy with several patients.

Patients in today's hospitals are sicker than they ever were before and patients are discharged faster than ever before. Patient care is described as "sicker and quicker," and that "efficiency" adds a unique challenge to the teaching process. When is the patient ready to learn? The nurse must diagnose the patient's problem and monitor the patient's response to their illness to know when the teachable moment is and how much teaching is appropriate at a given time.

The nurse teaches both the patient and the family. Although students hear in class that the "patient" is considered to be both the individual and the family, they tell me they are surprised when they are asked to explain the illness and the treatment to members of the family. Melinda wrote, "I wish that I knew that in pediatrics you're not just caring for a sick child but you are also caring for and listening to the concerns, troubles, and questions of their parents." Marie had an opportunity to teach both the patient and his wife:

I gathered the necessary pamphlets the unit has for patients and proceeded to see Mr. J around 10:00 A.M. As soon as he sees me at the door, he smiled and asked me to come in. I pulled a chair and sat beside the bed. I can see that he is prepared to listen to what I will say. I showed a picture of the heart and showed him where the stent was placed. I explained the reason why he needed the stent and what it will do after being placed there. I can see the interest in his face and proceeded to explain the pathophysiology of high blood pressure in layman's language. I kept on looking at his face and I can see slowly the lifting of the black veil. I advised him to do some lifestyle changes regarding work schedule and have more rest, diet emphasizing low sodium and low fat foods, and to exercise regularly. He admitted that he has to make a "big" change in order to live longer. He said, "I want to see my children grow into an adult and I will do anything to make that happen."

Towards the end of the teaching, his wife came in and I introduced myself to her. When I told her what I was doing there, she asked me to stay a little bit and explain everything to her again because she really want to get involved in her huband's health from now on. I explained everything to her starting from the diagram of the heart to the diet. She was appreciative of the teaching given and told me, " Thank you very much for enlightening me about this disease. I have nobody to talk with. I have been asking friends about heart conditions and they give me only bits and pieces. You made me understand what I need to know."

Hearing those words from a family member boosted my confidence in teaching people. I know that I don't need fancy English words to give my message across. I have been struggling with my communication skills since I started nursing school and I think I have improved a lot. I only need simple words that any non-medical person can understand. Educating a patient and family member and knowing that they understood it is a rewarding feeling. It gives them the information they need to make informed decisions about their health care treatments and knowledge to perform self-care. It gives me, on the other hand, confidence to speak and practice the English language.

The Diagnostic and Monitoring Function

When you think about what nurses do, it does not appear that nurses diagnose; that's the physician's job, right? Actually, nurses diagnose nursing problems. Nurses diagnose the patient's response to their illness, the patient's response to interventions, and the patient's response to medications. We already know about the nurse's role in the response to illness, right? The nurse also monitors treatment and medication responses. As Benner says, "Many diagnostic tests require careful monitoring, and the margins of safety are often narrow" (1984, p. 95). With new medications, the nurse must be aware of potential side effects and toxic levels. Not only does the nurse diagnose problems, but the nurse also anticipates problems and recognizes patient's needs.

The diagnostic and monitoring function consists of:

1. detection of changes in condition
2. anticipating problems
3. anticipating patient needs
4. assessing the potential for wellness or death with dignity.

October, a nurse returning for her Bachelor's degree, entitled her narrative "Life Preserver," which aptly communicates her role with this patient:

I understand the disease process, but my primary focus is the patient. It is my job to look outside of the box of the ICU, the constant flow of patients and doctors in and out, the invasive procedures at the bedside, the focus on tests to evaluate the patient's condition: CT scans, X-rays, and labs. I embrace my duty to understand the patient, his history, perception of his current condition, and how each element influences the present moment and his future.

I connect to the patient, the human being that has existed longer than the illness, by making eye contact and human contact through touch and by listening. As the wife left for the daughter's awards ceremony, these were the skills I depended on when the patient looked at me with the picture of death in his eyes, his deep dark pupils opening the door to his weary soul as he remarked, "I'm not going to make it through this, am I?" I felt time stop. I stopped what I was doing and placed the tangled IV tubing on the bedside table. Letting go of the tasks that so often consume our time, I observed this man in this moment, as I thought to myself, "No, you're not." Instead of responding with words of false hope, I placed my right hand on his, my left hand on his shoulder, and I acknowledged his concern; his water-filled eyes displayed a fear of what was to come. I empathized with the patient, "This is difficult for you," to which he responded with a confirming nod and downward gaze.

As an experienced nurse of seven years, I have come to respect the patient's ability to sense things such as death, and my sense was that the patient was correct. Although I could carry out orders that would keep his blood pressure within normal limits or administer meds to promote electrolyte balance, I recognized that I could not ensure that he would attend his daughter's graduation or meet his new grandchild. My job was to provide comfort, alleviate his anxieties, and provide him with distractions from the intense environment of the unit.

I assisted Mr. C. in finding a position of comfort, elevating his edematous legs on pillows. I massaged his feet with Sleepy Time lavender lotion and obtained an order for his usual bedtime Ativan, a ritual at home. I rolled the unit television into his room and turned on the Red Sox game, listening as he reminisced about their recent World Series success.

October reflects, "These are not skills that you can read about in a book or study; these are the true characteristics of nurses. I was not a lifesaver today, but a preserver of human dignity, and for that the family thanked me."

The nurse attended to the patient's illness by monitoring his body's response while she remained attentive and present with the whole patient.

The nurse must think on her feet and manage conditions that may change rapidly. With her knowledge and experience, the nurse decides when to page the physician, when to call in the social worker, or when to bring in the chaplain.

Effective Management of Rapidly Changing Conditions

This includes:

1. rapid grasp of the problem
2. rapidly matching needs and resources
3. identifying and managing crisis until the physician arrives

Danuta describes an emergent, rapidly changing condition, when she had to think on her feet to save the patient:

I was covering my fellow RN for lunch break when I heard a telemetry alarm go off. At the same time, I heard someone scream. I started running toward the room where the noise was coming from. In the background, I could here someone yelling, "Check on 45a, Mr. Smith is having Torsades!" I knew what Torsades meant: a ventricular tachycardia typically caused by medication or electrolyte imbalances. If not treated, it could cause ventricular fibrillation and cardiac arrest, a lethal electrical storm inside the heart, often resulting in the absence of a pulse and imminent death.

As I ran into the room, I could see Mr. Smith's whole body jump. He was a 50-year-old male dressed in a hospital jonnie sitting in a blue recliner chair with his legs elevated. His skin was pale and sweaty; he had a grim on his face that could only mean one thing, "I'm in pain." This was confirmed by his loud screams and swears. Within seconds I realized what was happening; his defib-rillator was firing. When defibrillator fires, it delivers a large amount of electric-ity to the heart. It "stuns" the heart muscle; allows for depolarization and resumption of normal activity by the heart. The patient feels the electricity shock; it is a very painful experience. Mr. Smith's heart was in trouble. I could feel adrenaline rush throughout my body, my heart was pounding, and my cheeks got red—my heart was experiencing a little storm of its own. It was my typical reaction to an emergency. I have been a nurse for three years. I'm expe-rienced in cardiology and know what to do when my patient's heart goes into arrhythmia. However, I still get the same adrenaline rush. I feel panic just like during my first code. I wanted to save this patient! Can I do it? I knew I needed to stay calm. I took a deep breath and got to my patient's bedside.

Mr. Smith was awake and alert but very agitated and upset. I explained what just happened and assured him I was there to help. Within seconds, my fellow coworkers ran into the room. It became loud and crowded. I delegated to the nursing assistant to help Mr. Smith's roommate out of the room. I designated one of my fellow RNs to page the patient's physician stat; I asked another nurse to page IV therapy to access another line. We needed another IV access to supply his body with IV medications that would calm the electrical storm booming inside his heart.

I checked Mr. Smith's blood pressure and reassessed his neurological status. He was feeling better, but still little upset about what had just happened. His physician was calling me back. I designated one of the nurses to stay with Mr. Smith while I took this phone call. In concise words, I explained what had just happened. He answered, "Give 2 mg of Magnesium in 50 cc of D5W over 10 minutes, start Lidocaine drip at 4 mg/minute and Amiodarone bolus 150 mg IV over 10 minutes, and then continue infusion at 17 cc/hr." I wrote his orders on paper and read them back to him. In a back of my mind I was thinking how glad I was that I requested the extra IVs to be started. "I will be right there," the physician stated and hung up the phone. I was relieved to know that he was on his way to see this patient.

Since I needed to start three different medications drips, I asked my fellow nurses for help to speed up the process. Everyone was rushing, getting IV tubing, mixing medications with IV solutions, double-checking orders, medication doses and compatibilities as well as drip rates—all of these procedures are done to assure the patent's safety. Meanwhile, nursing assistants were rechecking the patient's blood pressure, looking for IV pumps, and keeping Mr. Smith's roommate calm.

*I explained to Mr. Smith what was happening; we were starting all of these dif-
ferent drips to prevent his heart from going back into Torsades. Within minutes,
drips were infusing and a physician was at the patient's bedside. Mr. Smith was
stable now, his heart was slowing down, and he looked more comfortable. I could
feel my body relax, my heartbeat was slowing down too.*

Danuta made the diagnosis, responded to the problem, delegated
responsibilities to her team, and called in the physician, all in a matter of
moments.

Administering and Monitoring Interventions by Ensuring Quality and Safety

Tanya managed to administer and monitor interventions and ensure
safety:

*I entered the well-lit room with concern on my mind and probably on my
face. Michael was lying in the bed supine with the head of the bed inclined
30 degrees. He was balding. His face was red, he had beads of sweat on his
forehead and chest, and he was shaking rigorously. He was looking at me like
a deer caught in headlights. His eyes were the size of pancakes. Fear was written all over his face. My heart was heavy. I knew I needed to assess the situation and help him fast. I asked him how he was feeling. He stated he had a
headache and asked if I could turn the lights off. I assured him I would turn
the lights off after I was able to assess him. I looked at his flow sheet, checked
his incision and pedal pulse. His blood pressure was 186/110, temperature
101.6, heart rate 120; there was no evidence of bleeding or hematoma at the
incision and pedal pulses were palpable. I proceeded to my second inclination
and asked if he was having any chest and/or abdominal discomfort or short-
ness of breath. He stated "No." I obtained a 12 lead EKG, which showed no
depressions or elevations of the ST segments. This would be an indication of
lack of oxygen or blood supply to his heart and/or restenosis of the newly
placed stent. I had essentially ruled out hemodynamic instability as evidenced
by the above assessments. The only other obvious reason for his symptoms I
could explain was withdrawal from alcohol.*

*Due to the severity of his symptoms, I knew I should act fast. I asked Michael if
he drank alcohol. He looked away from me and stated, "Sometimes." I proceeded
to sit down next to him, smile and say, "Michael, it is important that you are
honest with me regarding your drinking. I am not here to judge you. In order for*

me to care for you and prevent you from having a seizure, this information is important." You could see the muscles in his face relax. He turned his head toward me and stated that he was a daily drinker since he was 18 and currently drank 8 to 10 hard liquor drinks daily. I questioned him regarding the last time he had a drink and he said it had been the evening before around 8:00 P.M.

This was important to track what stage of withdrawal he was experiencing and how quickly his symptoms may progress. I thanked him for his honesty, turned the lights out, gave him his call bell, and assured him I would return after speaking with the physician.

I paged the physician, who called back immediately. I reviewed my findings with the physician. A Clinical Institute Withdrawal Assessment for Alcohol (CIWA), a tool to monitor and stage symptoms of withdrawal, was initiated. To prevent seizure and diminish symptoms, benzodiazepines were administered. The physician also requested that blood and urine cultures be obtained to rule out sepsis and/or infection, a complete blood count and troponin level be drawn to rule out internal bleed, and postprocedure myocardial infarction and 5 mg IV lopressor, a beta blocker, be given now and in 1 hour to assist with decreasing heart rate and blood pressure. Furthermore, an IV bag of saline with multivitamin, folic acid, and thiamine was ordered to infuse to assist with nutritional deficiencies that often accompany alcoholism.

Tanya's knowledge of the science of illness, her relationship with the patient, and her collaboration with the physician brought Michael to safety. Tanya was competent and organized in her approach. Organization is an essential nursing skill.

Organizational Competencies

Organizational competencies consist of:

1. coordinating, prioritizing, and meeting multiple needs of the patient
2. building and maintaining a therapeutic team

In this case, Mary coordinated multiple needs of the patient and family as well as built and maintained a therapeutic team:

My patient was diagnosed with end-stage metastatic lymphoma. She was in excruciating pain with only days to live. Our pain service was called in for consult. The patient's family begged us to give her anything to stop her agonizing screams. She was already on high dose dilaudid intravenously and was suffering the side effect of myoclonic seizures. After consulting with multiple attending physicians managing the case and consulting with hospital administration, the decision was made to initiate a propofol infusion on a standard nursing unit. This was the first time a sedative/hypnotic agent was used in a noncritical care area of the hospital. Under the supervision of the anesthesiologists, the infusion was started and titrated for her comfort. The patient grabbed my arm and thanked me. Then she closed her eyes. Her family surrounded her at the bedside and was relieved at the ceasing of her screams. I stayed on beeper call for 24 hours, coming in during the night to adjust the medicine to maintain her level of comfort. After three days of ease with her family, she was able to die a peaceful, painless, dignified death.

Mary reflects, "I have learned that at times no invasive interventions may be the best treatment."

To manage this case, the nurse had to conduct a thorough assessment of the patient by knowing her history and understanding the disease process. The nurse listened to the needs of the family, related the story to the physician, met with the anesthesiologist to develop a new procedure, and then she volunteered for 24-hour call to implement the procedure. In the midst of all the action, Mary maintained a presence for the patient and her family.

Reflection 2: Take-Home Message

What is the take-home message from this chapter?

What information was new to you?

The different roles of the nurse give you more of an idea of what you will do as a nursing student and as a practicing nurse. What do you think? Still interested in nursing? In the next chapter, we will look closer at how your expectations fit with nursing.

CONCLUSION

In this first chapter, we dove right in to learning what nurses actually do, how nurses think, and what it is like to work in different specialties. A central aspect of the chapter was going behind the closed doors into the world of patient care. The nurse narratives give a good sense of what kinds of patients nurses work with and how much nurses need to know to perform their roles. Nursing is definitely an exciting place to be! In Chapter 2, we will assess your fit with nursing.

END-OF-CHAPTER EXERCISE

Find out as much as you can about nursing. You are choosing your life's work and preparing to compete for selective, rigorous programs. Find out about the important issues in health care and in nursing. Gather as much information as possible. Conduct your own investigation by consulting with your own sources to learn more about the inside story of nursing:

1. Does someone in your family or a friend know a nurse? Don't be shy about contacting a nurse. Nurses love to talk about their profession.

2. Review nursing web sites:
   http://www.nursema.org/
   http://www.massnurses.org/
   http://www.nursingworld.org

3. Rent the film *Wit* which is a brilliant depiction of the nurse, patient, and physician relationship. All students recommend this film.

4. Read a book about a day in the life of a nurse:
   a. Gordon, S. (1997). *Life Support.* New York: Little Brown & Co.
   b. Heron, E. (1987). *Intensive Care.* New York: Ivy Books.
   c. Banks, J. T., Davis, C. and Schaefer, J. (1995). *Between the heart beats: Poetry and Prose by Nurses.* New York: Random House.
   d. Davis, C. (2001). *I Knew a woman.* New York: Random House.
   e. Lascala, S. (2007). *Small wonder.* MA: Haley's Publishing.

5. Pay attention to local and global health issues on the news, and in magazines and newspapers.

6. Go to your local college library and thumb through professional nursing journals or visit the journal web sites:

   a. American Journal of Nursing: http://www.ajn.com.

   b. Nursing 2007 magazine.

7. Talk to a nurse.

   a. Ask about alums of the program you are looking into

   b. Go to your local hospital human resources department and ask about how to meet a nurse. Don't be shy about this. You will be welcomed with open arms. Everyone needs nurses, especially nurses who ask questions.

References

Benner, P. (1984). *From novice to expert.* CA: Addison-Wesley Publishing Company.

Henderson, V. (1966). *The nature of nursing: A definition and its implications for practice, research, and education.* New York: Macmillan.

CHAPTER 2

How Do I Get There from Here?

What Is Nursing School Like?

Nursing school is as exciting, demanding, and challenging as nursing practice. Nursing, in fact, is like no other college major. As a nursing student, you are not just taking classes, writing papers, and doing research; you also are applying knowledge and learning skills on real patients in real hospitals. There is a T-shirt that says "Nursing is a kind, compassionate, and rewarding profession. Nursing School is cruel and unusual punishment." I won't lie to you, according to our students, some days with classes and practicing in the hospital, the nursing major does feel overwhelming. I remember those early clinical days . . .

Picture this: You are living in a dorm with friends who are majoring in sociology, political science, and psychology. These students start classes at noon and sometimes only have one class a day. Your friends are out partying all night coming in at 4:30 A.M. Now that is college, right? You, as a nursing major, just as your friends are pulling in at 4:30 A.M., you are getting up at 4:30 A.M. to get ready to go to the hospital. When I was in college, this scene alone caused me to question my decision to major in nursing. In fact, I went so far to talk to alumni to see if I shouldn't transfer to another major. Their response was one line: "You're the only one that'll have a job when you graduate." I did stick it out and they were right. I moved to Boston to be a nurse and my three college roommates, the soc, poly sci and psych major, moved with me to be waitresses. So, yes, it is hard work to become a nurse, but no other major can compare to the rich experience of a nursing student.

Nursing is a unique major. To help you prepare for entering this intense area of study, we will visit students who are in nursing programs now and we will hear what they wish someone had told them, so that you will feel better prepared for your college adventure.

Most college students ease into freshman year with classes of their choice, a bit of studying, and a lot of socializing. You are expected to manage your course workload and your extracurricular activities and to make new friends all at the same time. But, hey, it looks like there is plenty of time compared to the eight hours a day you were locked away in high school. Typically, first-year students choose their own classes in which they are assigned books to read, articles to research, homework assignments, papers to write, and a mid-term and final exam. Nursing is different. Students who major in nursing start first semester with a *prescribed* list of classes that require a sophisticated understanding of difficult subjects, volumes of reading, and an intense amount of memorization for the frequent quizzes and challenging exams. Although prenursing students are told that chemistry and microbiology will lay the groundwork for the nursing classes and they will provide you with a base for your work with patients, it can be difficult to envision being at the bedside when you are bogged down with four chapters in the micro-book. The fact is, anatomy, microbiology, and pathophysiology will relate to medical nursing, pediatric nursing, and mental health nursing. For example, nursing students must know how the lungs function to know how to care for a patient with pneumonia, microbiology comes into play when learning about the disease process of a bacterial infection, and chemistry will assist you in understanding fluid and electrolyte balance. Make sense? The prenursing courses prepare you for your role as health care provider. One student wrote:

I had no idea I would be on my own so fast as a nursing student. I did not picture having my own patients. Somehow I thought I'd be washing patients, comforting them, giving medication already prepared. I did not know I would have to know the medication, calculate the dosage and teach the patient about the medication and the side effects. I figured I'd assist the real nurses. But now I have my own patients. I pictured the doctors being around and they would be helpful. But I may not even see the doctor. They will just come in and write an order then I have to make it happen. The good thing is the nurse is much more independent than I thought. That is also the scary thing.

By junior year, while other friends are in class focusing on topics specific to their major, nursing students are not only studying pharmacology for a medication quiz but they are studying the night before they go to the hospital to be prepared to give an injection of the medication they just memorized. In addition, students must know how to translate the complex information they have learned about the medication to teach the patient and their family about the drug's intended action and the possible side effects. Nursing students are out in the work world before any other students on campus.

Like other college students, nursing students are learning how to conduct research on topics in their major so that they can write the required papers. However, in addition to writing papers, nursing students research topics that are real problems in the clinical setting, such as the effects of domestic violence on the patient they took care of last week who had two broken hands and a black eye. Other majors are writing papers about a possible future career. Nursing students have the opportunity to read and write about topics they are dealing with in their clinical experience that day.

Despite all the tempting diversions in college, prenursing students have to become serious students their very first semester to maintain the required grade point average (GPA) to be admitted into the nursing program. Currently, there are at least two types of admission processes in 4-year schools. That is, some schools admit prenursing students in their freshman year to the university and then the student has to compete and apply for limited positions in the nursing school during their sophomore year. Some schools admit you directly into the nursing program. Make sure that you read the fine print so that you know which program you are applying for. There are advantages to each admission policy. If you are admitted right into the nursing major then you would have had to know in high school that nursing was your choice of major. If you are admitted as a prenursing student you have a chance to get to college, take a few classes and then decide if you want to apply to nursing. In schools that have a prenursing program there is a chance you will not be admitted into the nursing major. Then you would have to transfer majors, wait to try again for admission or transfer to another school with a nursing major.

All nursing students are required to maintain a higher GPA than other majors. Katelyn writes:

The first time I heard the GPA that I was going to need to get into the program I almost had a heart attack. I thought there was no way I could get grades that were that good. But, as it turns out college is very different from high school. Once I began taking classes that interested me the work became less tedious. I found myself saying less and less, "when am I ever going to use this?" but rather now I am saying, "I am going to use all of this. How can I remember it all?"

Dan, a student at a large University, acknowledges,

From the beginning I was working harder and had a higher GPA than some of my friends.

Listen in on what Megan, a junior student, advises:

Coming from high school to college is a huge transition, especially when you choose nursing as a major. Not everyone understands the focus that is necessary to be successful in this major. Making friends within the major as well as having outside friends is a necessity, however, the realization that social activities is not always a possibility needs to be known. Peer pressure is huge on the weekend but as a nursing major the opportunity for a social life is not always possible.

Deciding to apply to a nursing program means deciding to become a serious student with perseverance, motivation, and commitment. Before investing your time, effort, and money in a program, make sure majoring in nursing is the right choice for you.

Reflection 1

Take a moment to respond to the following questions. The answers will begin to assist you in deciding how you fit with nursing.

• What started you thinking about nursing as a career? Just jot a few ideas down:

_____

_____

• What attracted you to nursing? Write down the answer that first comes to mind:

_____

_____

• I want to be a nurse because:

_____

_____

_____

_____

Do any of your reasons for looking into nursing compare to the reasons prenursing students give for deciding to become a nurse? Students say that they chose nursing for five primary reasons:

1. Nursing is inherited

2. Nursing is caring

3. Nursing is exciting

4. Nursing makes a difference

5. Nursing is a science

Nursing Is Inherited

I've always known I wanted to be a nurse. When I was a little girl my aunt would stop by after her shift and regale us with her funny, sad, heroic stories. I knew that was just what I wanted to do when I grew up.

Students report that they want to be a nurse because their favorite aunt has been a pediatric nurse for years and they always knew they would grow up to be a nurse. It seems like half of all the nursing applicants are related to a nurse. Nursing was in their genes. Val writes about her path to nursing:

My mother was a nurse, her three sisters were nurses, and just about any woman in the community with a financially stable job was a nurse. I wanted to be different, to make a difference. As time was passing by and the years out of high school increasing, it was time to choose a focus. What could one in the

Berkshires do? According to a close friend at the time, nursing paid well and supported continuing education. The prospect of getting a job out of school was guaranteed. This is exactly what happened in 1999 when I graduated from Berkshire Community College with an Associate's degree in Nursing.

For some, nursing is inherited, for others, caring comes naturally.

Nursing Is Caring

Everyone comes to me with their problems. All my friends confide in me, I help my parents and brother sort out their differences. I am a good listener. I think I would be a good nurse.

Every year, I ask the new freshman class why they want to major in nursing. The answer is always, "Because I want to take care of people." New students see themselves as caring individuals who have a natural fit with nursing. With the realities of the lives of our patients, experience with personal caring provides a good base for professional caring. As a nursing professor, I want to build on student's passion to care for others but I also want eager, bright-eyed students to be aware of what they are getting themselves into, so I wrote this poem:

These novice students picture delivering healthy babies, They cuddle the child in the pediatric intensive care that is not too sick, just cute.

They see themselves in the ER where no one dies or in Cardiac Care where the middle-aged man welcomes the ministrations of the nurse.

They know the cachetic woman slumped in a chair on the Alzheimer's unit will notice their soft touch.

They want to make a difference.

They don't know they will be the one who changes.

The babies they help deliver will be from 14 year old mothers with Hep C

With no father in sight.

The children in the Pedi ICU are very sick and cranky and pale and thin and dying.

The trauma in the ER is wheeled out in a body bag.

The man with the heart attack is so angry he was struck down

He yells at anyone who walks into his room,

And our Alzheimer's lady never . . . even . . . moves.

Being a caring person is a good start, but it is only the beginning. Caring in nursing is different than caring for your little brother or your best friend. Nursing involves professional care that is developed with knowledge, experience, and a good sense of who you are. Professional caring enables you to take care of all types of patients with different kinds of illnesses in a variety of settings. No two patients will be alike. Each patient will require a different approach. The unique needs of individual patients, with their own response to their illness, is what make nursing a rich and varied career choice.

Nursing Is Exciting

I am an adrenalin junky and I get this rush from staying on the brink of being overwhelmed and riding this powerful wave through the situation. This is very important in my job working as a paramedic and will be important to me as a nurse.—Peter

The nurses in ER are ready for anything that walks through the door. From jumping into the life flight helicopter to pounding on a patient's chest, nurses in real life *are* in the middle of the action. The difference between Hollywood and real life is the adventures in the Emergency Room do not stop after a 60-minute program. In real life, after 60 minutes the nurse is on duty for the next 11 hours on the 7 P.M. to 7 A.M. shift. You are on your feet for 11 hours, that is, if you get off your shift on time. Then, unlike the once-a-week show, you are back the next night for another 12 hours. There is no question nursing can be exciting but the work is also demanding. Both the excitement and the demand are rewarding because nurses impact people's lives.

Nursing Makes a Difference

I've been a software engineer for 20 years. Now I want to have more of a direct impact on people's lives.—Vanessa

Nurses definitely have an impact on people's lives. Nurses work 24/7, the nurse is the provider most directly involved with the patient. The nurse recognizes changes in an illness or anticipates a response to treatments, the nurse coaches the patient and teaches the family, they decide when to intervene, when to call the physician and when to wait and see, just as nursing student, Jill, did:

Lela was unusually drowsy and sedated. Her speech was slurred and she would fall asleep mid-sentence and doze off with a spoon in her hand while eating. Her excessive drowsiness concerned me and I searched for an explanation. In reviewing her medication profile I noticed that Lela was prescribed three medications to control her blood pressure to keep it from rising while she was withdrawing from alcohol. As I reviewed her history I noticed she did not have a history of high blood pressure. This combination of drugs could be a possible explanation for her drowsiness . . . and Jill proceeded to consult with the physician who was unaware of the patient's medication cocktail.

Lela, the patient in the story, is fortunate to have a thorough, inquisitive nursing student who does not accept the first response, "Oh, this is just the way she is." But, rather, Jill searched further for an explanation of the patient's condition. Jill's commitment to her patient and her critical thinking on the topic of drug interactions enabled her to become a bridge between the patient and the physician. Nurses are on the front line, providing caring that is based on the science of nursing.

Nursing Is a Science

I was attracted to the nursing major because I was good in science and math but I did not want to work in a lab. I wanted hands-on.

Nursing builds on chemistry, microbiology, anatomy, and physiology. Nursing will give you the opportunity to apply science with real people in real settings. Nursing research forms the evidence base on which nurses build their practice. For example, the research that Cheryl Beck, DNSc, CNM, FAAN, has conducted on postpartum depression helps the nurse provide better care for patients and their families. See the references at the end of the chapter for journals that have published the results of Dr. Beck's research.

Nursing science, a lifelong ambition, wanting to make a difference, and a caring nature are all good reasons to pursue a career in nursing. There are also many advantages of a career in nursing.

NURSING AS A CAREER

Some students decide to go into nursing because of all the job opportunities. What about the job is appealing to you? With the global need for nurses, nursing is a guaranteed lifelong career that is mobile and flexible. Think about the career flexibility in nursing—a flexible schedule, career mobility, and a challenging patient assignment every day—how good does it get?

Flexible Schedule

In some hospitals, you can work for 8 hours from 7 to 3, 3 to 11, or 11 to 7. You can work 12 hours, 3 or 4 days a week from 7 A.M. to 7 P.M. Hospitals are open 24/7. You can work 24/7 if you'd like. The schedule flexibility can work for a nurse. The 3–11 shift was ideal for me when I first graduated. Because all my sociology and psychology friends were now waitresses working 4–11, we could all go to the beach in the morning and meet up after work. Later in my life, with a family, the 7–3 shift fit better. Some nurses choose different shifts because the activity on each shift varies so much. On the day shift, there are more providers around, patients are scheduled for exams, lab work, and X-rays. In the evening, those departments close, social workers, physicians, and physical therapists all go home, families come in to visit, and the nurse runs the show. On the night shift, it is all nursing.

Joullen has worked on the oncology night shift for 15 years. "At night these are all my patients. I wouldn't have it any other way."

The flexible schedule can also work against the individual nurse. All the units need to be covered; days, nights, and weekends, which mean nurses need to work days, nights, and weekends.

- What if you have worked a 7–3 shift and someone calls in sick on the next shift and the central office asks you to stay another 8 hours, but you have to pick up the kids and have dinner plans? What about your life?
- What if you worked all night and were asked to stay on days? What happens to the dentist appointment you had waited 6 months for?

What about your book club meeting that night or your bike-riding plans?

- If you refuse to work what happens to your patients? How are your colleagues going to manage with fewer staff? What about *their* lives?

Flexible schedules can work for you and they can work against you. The nursing staff should have a say in staffing; you should inquire about mandatory overtime policies before taking a job.

Mobility

Nursing jobs are mobile. You can move from one specialty to another. Within one organization you can go from Labor & Delivery to the OR, from the OR to the day-stay surgery unit. You can move from providing bedside care in a hospital to providing nursing care in a home through a visiting nurse association. You can travel across the country working for an agency (Google "travel nurse") or travel around the world working for an international group. As your needs change, your job can change. In the early part of your career, moving around is appealing. Later, when you are more settled, staying in one place may be attractive. Then, after the kids are grown, mobility may have a pull again. That's the good news.

Sometimes, however, mobility is not your idea. The organization you are working for wants you to be mobile and that is not at all what you had planned. You arrive to work on your usual ICU unit and you are told to go to the ER because they are short-staffed. That can work once or twice, but if floating to another unit is not your decision, then floating does not work for long. Moving to different units and working with staff you do not know may not be comfortable or safe, for that matter. Flexibility and mobility can work for or against you during a career that can be lifelong. We now have three generations working together in nursing, the new 20- to 30-year-old nurse, the mid-level 30- to 60-year-old nurse, and the senior, 60- to 75-year-old nurse. You can be a nurse from graduation to retirement and even after retirement choose to work part time!

A Lifelong Career

A career for your entire life in a demanding profession sounds good, but nursing could drain the life right out of you (which is probably why there is such a high attrition rate). Unless you are able to manage your career with equanimity and balance by finding the work environment that matches your expectations, values, and ambitions, and you are able to maintain a fulfilling outside life and have a good support base, you may experience burnout.

In a study of expert nurses my friend flew out to San Francisco to interview those nurses who were nominated "experts" by their colleagues. The problem was she could never find these experts to conduct an interview with. The expert nurse was either working a 12-hour shift with not a minute to stop and chat or not working and out of town. When she finally did figure out how to corral the expert nurse, the results of her study revealed that part of being a expert nurse was taking care of yourself so when you were working you could provide the focus and critical thinking necessary for expertise. Skipping town on each day off was part of the reason the nurse was able to develop into an expert: when they were not working they were taking care of themselves, doing something fun, getting outside, visiting friends, getting far away from their work environment. When they returned to work they were refreshed and ready to go.

Actually, most jobs will own you if you do not find a balance between work and play. But working with sick people in vulnerable situations tends to make those in the service professions more susceptible to burnout. Burnout isn't necessarily bad. In fact, there is a saying, "You can't burn out if you have never been on fire." And our current health system definitely needs on-fire nurses! Burnout is actually only a symptom that lets you know that something is out of balance in your professional life or your personnel life or between your work and your outside life. The feeling of exhaustion that burnout brings is asking you to slow down and reflect on what is going on. We nurses like action, so sometimes it takes a case of burnout to slow us down and take a breath. Exhaustion offers us an opportunity, a time to sit back and look at how we schedule our lives. With the intense work of nursing, it is critical to manage your career and understand the role of burnout. The same skills are required to managing your student career and protect you from burnout during your school days. Taking care of yourself is the key in school and in practice. In the meantime, it is important to note that each asset to working as a nurse, flexibility, mobility, and life career, has its own liability (Table 2-1).

Does this type of job fit in your future? Which type of nursing program will get you where you want to go?

Table 2-1. Summary of assets and liabilities regarding length of career, flexibility of schedule, and mobility

Nursing career	Assets	Liabilities
Lifelong career	Excitement, challenge	Every shift is exciting and challenging = exhaustion
Flexible schedule	A varied schedule to meet your needs	A varied schedule to meet organizational needs
Mobility	Many different specialties to choose from	Many different specialties required within one week

NURSING PROGRAMS

Fortunately, there are several paths to becoming a registered nurse. In all programs, you will be in the classroom setting for part of the time, practicing skills in a nursing lab and out in a clinical setting learning how to apply the classroom knowledge and the laboratory skills with real patients. In the classroom you will learn about aspects of nursing from pharmacology to developmental theories. During class there will be an opportunity to review your findings from your reading, discuss your opinions, and analyze your experience with classmates. Much of the learning will take place outside of class through reading texts and researching current nursing literature, writing papers, and working on group projects. There will be required presentations, public speaking, and group work. Students are expected to be prepared to participate in class and perform during clinical in each of the different nursing programs.

With the competition to get into nursing school all possible avenues for entering nursing should be researched. Many of the programs build on each other. Some nurses begin as a licensed practical nurse (LPN) and move into an associate degree (AD) program. Others start at the community college and receive a 2-year AD in nursing. Once you have your AD, you can take the registered nurse (RN) licensing exam and begin to work or you may choose to go right on to a baccalaureate (BS) degree program. For the community college graduate, there are many RN to BS programs on line or in-person that can be completed in a year. Some students decide to start out majoring in nursing at a 4-year college or university. And still others complete their 4-year bachelors degree in another major, work for a while, and then return to earn a nursing degree in a second bachelor's program. Confused? You are not the only one. Take some time to review the possibilities to make sure you choose the program that fits your career goals. Here is the inside story on nursing programs.

Licensed Practical Nurse

A Licensed Practical Nurse (LPN) program or Licensed Vocational Nurse (LVN) program is about a year long and offered at vocational or technical schools. At the end of the formal educational program you take a licensing exam. In practice, the LPN functions under the direction of a registered nurse providing basic care such as taking blood pressures, bathing patients, monitoring input and output, and changing dressings. To move to a RN position, you must return to school. Several community college programs offer advanced placement opportunities for LPNs.

Associate Degree in Nursing

To sit for the registered nurse license exam, one must have a degree from a hospital diploma program, an associate degree program, or a baccalaureate program. Historically, many nurses received a diploma from a hospital program. Today, in many parts of the country, diploma programs are being phased out or combined with community college AD programs. An associate degree is offered at a 2-year community college or as a 2-year program within a college or university. The typical AD program consists of classroom experience and clinical practice. The four semesters include basic and advanced medical-surgical nursing, maternal-newborn, pediatrics, mental health, and a leadership or community course. An AD graduate can sit for the RN licensing exam to become a registered nurse. An AD nurse can give direct patient care in most settings. However, some specialty branches of nursing require a BS degree.

Associate Degree to Baccalaureate Degree: RN to BS

Why go back to school? You are an expert in your nursing practice, why add the burden of school? There are three types of responses to the nagging "why go back?" question:

1. "I have to. My hospital is pushing us to be baccalaureate prepared."
2. "I want to. I feel like there in so much to learn to give good patient care."
3. "I need more. I recognize there is more to nursing than what I am doing and I want to advance my career."

The "I have to" student is the one who sits in the back of the room, slouched down in those compact chairs with the little attached desk surface. Their arms are crossed tightly over their chest and they have the look of "What are you, Miss PhD, possibly going to teach me, The Captain of the ER?" I love these challenges and admit right away that the students bring their clinical expertise to the classroom and I have some research, leadership and theory expertise that we can combine and come up with a worthwhile product. In the end we are all working well together. The "I want to" student has always loved learning and recognizes as health care becomes more complex so do their learning needs. More education is inevitable. The "I need more" student is a bit bored with their current role and would like to expand their knowledge base to fulfill their desire for learning. They have specialty certification and attend continuing education programs but have that gnawing sense that there must be more. Time to go back to school.

Many RNs enter college the same time that their kids do (see Chapter 5, "non-traditional student," for a good description of what returning to school is like as an adult). You, too, will have to arrange work and family to accommodate your study requirements. School cannot be just an "add-on." It doesn't work that way. The good news is you will meet many more people like you in the program and develop a new support group that will have solutions to the problems you are trying to figure out. One problem is likely to be the fear of putting yourself in the position of a student again. You have status and are recognized for your knowledge and skills. In school, students do not have much status and their knowledge base is challenged. Just like graduate students, returning RNs are likely to experience the imposter syndrome: "Am I smart enough to go to college?" See Chapter 7 for a thorough discussion of the imposter syndrome. You may recognize yourself. Fortunately today, there are several types of returning

RN programs that attend to the unique needs of the nontraditional student's commitment to education, work, and family. Choose the program that fits you.

Associate degree graduates have several choices to complete their baccalaureate degree. There are evening and weekend programs offered at your local college, partial online programs that have some Web-based instruction and some in-person time, and the full online, asynchronous programs that are offered at many schools. I know you may be thinking, "All online? How does that work?" Or "All online, impossible! I need the face-to-face contact." I know, because I felt the same way. I love teaching returning RNs. They are so committed to their careers and to furthering their education. As practicing nurses they have such great experience to bring into the classroom discussion. I learn from the returning nurses and they learn from me. Knowing the complexity of patient care and the need for well-educated providers, I am committed to nurses furthering their education. I have literally gone the distance to teach returning RNs from flying 2 hours from Salt Lake City to the middle of the desert to teach a weekend course to driving 2 hours out to the Berkshire Mountains in Massachusetts to a satellite university site at the community college. I initiated one of the first interactive video programs to enable BS education to meet the needs of working/family RNs. From the western desert to the eastern mountains, I loved being in class with the returning RNs. So how could I possibly work in an online environment? I was so critical of the notion of online learning that I volunteered to teach, "Writing and Ethics", class online to demonstrate that it could not be done. I worked hard to learn the online platform, to develop class content that would be interactive yet not require students to all be online at the same time and to create online resources that were easily accessible to students. Asynchronous learning is where students can sign into class anytime that is convenient for them. Sounds perfect for a working family-oriented nurse, yet many students were as reluctant as I was. In fact, many don't even consider the possibility of online education because they do not believe they will be able to learn without being in the classroom, nor are they confident in their computer skills. Some students that come into our program are just purchasing their first computer. Many rely on their teenagers for tech support. Most of us come in leery of what we were getting ourselves into. And guess what? Despite all the fears, my Writing online class worked. It worked well! I got to know every student and they got to interact one-on-one with the professor and each other. We knew each other better than we would have in person. And the student outcomes were better than in an in-person class. Every single student, from the 52-year-old computer averse to the second-language student, every student, became a better writer and every student increased their awareness and critical thinking about ethical issues. Course evaluations were overwhelmingly positive. Denuta, an RN for 10 years, wrote,

As I look back at the beginning of the semester I am quite pleased with what I have accomplished. I had approached this class with a grain of worry in my writing abilities. However what I have learned throughout this semester is that first of all I can write, secondly, what I do not know I can learn, and finally, constructive criticism can help me become a better writer. I have learned to communicate my ideas more clearly, and explore my abilities as a creative writer. This class helped me develop critical thinking skills and ability to critique various types of writing in professional nursing. Writing in ethics also helped me to learn and explore difficult ethical dilemmas and encouraged me to think about my own values and beliefs.

Val, a veteran nurse, commented:

Overall, I am much more comfortable in the research arena and I am extremely pleased that I learned how to find the most accurate, peer-reviewed literature that I can use in my practice. This, above all, I found most helpful. It's been at my fingertips the whole time and I have used this information several times in my practice already this semester. I have enjoyed finding the answers to some questionable practices in the nursing profession and in my community and I cannot imagine a time, henceforth, when I will not take a more proactive approach. It has changed my practice and my outlook on my profession.

And Bina, a second-language student, said:

I feel much more confident in writing. I would never be afraid of taking any class that requires writing in a future. I am sure that I still need a lot of improvement. I believe that perfection comes with practice. This was the first time I attempted to write this much in quality, quantity, and variety in English language. I certainly felt it but it has definitely played important part in boosting my confidence and self-esteem.

When I went back and reviewed the course evaluations I had hoped to find comments on using the technology, but there were none. Not one tech comment out of 22 students. Considering the course comments, you can see how transparent the technology becomes. When the technology becomes transparent it means that using the technology is a success. Success means technology is not a barrier but a tool that promotes learning. I proved myself wrong about online learning. I have signed up every semester since. Think about trying an online class.

Whether you choose to return to school in an online format or in a in-person class you will meet both colleagues and faculty that will become friends and mentors. Your world of nursing will broaden and from what I have heard, you will be more satisfied with your career.

Bachelor's of Science Degree

The traditional baccalaureate degree (BS) is offered at 4-year colleges and universities. The BS is the most marketable degree and is required in several settings. The military requires a BS degree as well as school nursing, public health nursing, and forensic nursing. The BS degree provides the opportunity for the greatest career advancement. With a BS, one can apply to graduate school to become a nurse practitioner, nurse midwife, nurse anesthetist, or nurse educator. A Master's degree graduate can study for a doctoral degree (PhD), which is a research degree or a doctorate of nursing practice (DNP), a practice degree. There is more on advanced degrees in Chapter 7. But, before we get to graduate school, let's look a typical plan of study for a BS student.

The Path to a BS Degree

Many undergraduate programs are divided into lower division courses taken in freshman and sophomore year and then upper division courses taken in junior and senior year. Nursing is often an upper division major. What this means is you take prerequisite courses and general education courses during your first 2 years. Gen. eds. usually meet two to three times a week, Tuesdays or Thursdays or Monday, Wednesday, and Friday. The nursing program will recommend some of the general education courses such as a course in sociology and psychology so that you will be prepared to take care of all types of patients in all types of settings. Other gen. ed. courses are electives for the student to chose in any area that is of interest, from yoga to myths of the Middle Ages. First-year students should take advantage of having a free choice in coursework because as you progress toward nursing the coursework will be more prescribed.

In freshman year, there may be an introductory course to nursing. This course is a general overview of what nursing is all about. If you choose a large university the introductory course may have 100 to 200 students enrolled, all deciding whether nursing is the major for them. The introductory course is where you will meet other students who are interested in nursing. It is a great time to make friends and develop connections to students, the teaching assistants, and the nursing faculty. There are often guest speakers who are practicing nurses or faculty who present issues in their practice area or their research program. Candice, a junior, wrote:

I wish someone had told me that the students I was meeting in my pre-req courses would end up being valuable resources to me. I can see now that what we are learning will affect the life or death of a patient. Had I begun thinking like this in freshman year and working with colleagues, the first 2 years would have been much more enjoyable and I probably would have learned more.

During sophomore year, there are more prerequisites such as microbiology and pathophysiology. Students say they wish they knew how to manage their time and develop good study habits before they got to these courses. Stephanie writes:

Probably the most important thing is time management and organizational skills. I already feel like if I miss a beat it takes longer to make up stuff and get things in on time. I wish I had practiced more time management before I got to the nursing classes.

After the first 2 years of classes, students enter into the upper division nursing, where they will have both nursing specialty classes and what is called "clinicals." Let me explain.

The nursing courses consist of general courses and specialty courses. Every student must take both general and specialty courses. The general courses in the beginning of the nursing program are often called fundamentals in nursing. In the fundamentals course, you learn how to give basic physical and emotional care to a patient. You will learn how to give a bed bath, and how to take the vital signs of blood pressure, pulse, and respiration. The first semester you will learn how to do a head-to-toe physical assessment from listening to the lungs, finding the heart beat or learning the different bowel sounds while listening to the patient's concerns. There will be classes in the lab so you can practice giving a bed bath and listening to breathing sounds on a patient model. In the beginning classes, you will learn about common patient problems such as discomfort and pain management. You will learn communication techniques. You will explore your values, learn about professional values, ethical principles, and legal requirements.

The following semester there are specialty classes in maternal-newborn health, mental health, the care of children, and the care of the elderly. There will be courses in public health nursing and course about providing nursing in the community. In baccalaureate programs there is a course in nursing research, and courses may be offered in ethics, culture, aging, health policy, and public health.

With each course that is held in a classroom there is a matching course in a clinical setting where you put your classroom learning to use with real patients. Some examples of where you will work with patients in the clinical setting are acute care hospitals, rehabilitation hospitals, nursing homes, clinics, or patient homes. Figure 2-1 shows what a schedule may look like.

Depending on the location of your school the clinical placements could be next door at the medical center or 2 hours, yup, a 2-hour drive, out to a community hospital. To drive to a clinical placement at 7:00 A.M. that is 2 hours away you would have to get up at 4:30 A.M., at the latest. But students report having great clinical experiences in remote settings. I just want to let you know of all the possibilities!

Monday	Tuesday	Wednesday	Thursday	Friday	Saturday	Sunday
9–12 Pharmacology		9–12 Health Assessment 1–3 a two hour Lab	7:00–1:00 or 1:00–7:00 Clinical	7–1 or 1–7 Clinical	May have Clinical	May have Clinical
1:30–4:30 Fundamentals in Nursing	1:00–4:00 Writing in Nursing Ethics	4–6 Cultural Diversity and Illness				

Figure 2-1. Typical schedule for junior year in a bachelor of science in nursing program, involving courses and clinical work.

In the clinical setting you will be assigned your own patient and take care of that patient for the time you are in the facility. In the last hour of the shift there is usually a post conference to discuss the daily experience with your instructor and fellow students.

Each of the four semesters in the junior and senior year you will be in a theory class and a clinical placement. Some programs end with an internship where you are in a clinical placement with a nurse preceptor for 20–30 hours/week. This final intensive experience provides you with an opportunity to pull all your new knowledge and skills together and work under the supervision of a real nurse. An internship gives you a taste of the real world of work and some extra clinical experience in an area of your choice.

What Real Students Say

When I conducted a survey of 100 new nursing students, 75% of the respondents said they wish they were told how much work nursing school would be. Many students reported that they breezed through high school and got good grades. They, too, wrote that they had no idea that they would need to work so many hours and have to learn so much. Kate admits:

My senior year was pretty much a joke and I figured college was going to be a breeze. I never really had a lot of work in high school and still got all As. When I got to college it was a completely different ballgame.

Caitlin confesses:

If I had known how much work the program was I would have waited to get my second Bachelor's in nursing so I could have enjoyed the college experience more with less stress.

Most students, once they get their feet wet, feel like Heather:

Most of all I wish someone had told me that all the stress would be worth it when I walked into my first clinical and could feel the excitement rushing through my veins. And also that I had chosen the right career path and it really was so worth it!

That is the main reason why people out in the workforce come back to school for nursing: for the excitement, the opportunity to give direct patient care, and the possibility of making a difference in the world, one patient at a time.

Second Degree Programs

There are also several options for students that have a bachelor's degree in another field and are returning for a nursing degree. The returning student can choose a program that offers a second bachelor's, a direct entry master's, or a fast-track doctoral program.

In today's world, they say we will have three to four different careers. Nursing, as a second or third career, is one of the options. Except for a few unique programs, before the 1990s, those interested in a second career in nursing would have to start at the beginning at either a community college or in a traditional 4-year program. Today, there are abbreviated programs specifically designed to meet the needs of a second career student.

The second bachelor's program goes from a year to 2-years, often running all 12 months of the year. There are usually five to eight prerequisite courses, depending on the specific school. Programs offer basic nursing courses with all of the clinical components that are in a traditional 4-year program. However, because the second degree program is shorter than the traditional undergraduate program, classes and clinicals are condensed into a shorter time period. For example, our program begins in January with a 2-week all-day workshop on the introduction to nursing. In the traditional program, the introductory course is required in freshman year and is offered in a 3-hour/day a week class for a 14-week semester. Our second degree students complete their maternity and pediatric rotation the first summer session and the psychiatric mental health rotation the second half of the summer. Although these courses are condensed, they work quite well for the adult returning student. At the completion of the program the graduate is well prepared to sit for the RN licensing exam.

The second bachelor's students come from all walks of life: from the humanities, theater, biology, carpentry to computer programming. Some students are just out of college, others have been in the workforce for over 20 years. The combination of varied backgrounds, different work experience, and a wide student age range make the second bachelor's classes very interesting. The American Association of Colleges of Nursing

(AACN, 2004) reports, "The typical second degree student is motivated, older and has higher academic expectations . . . they excel in class . . . faculty find them excellent learners who are not afraid to challenge instructors." Faculty love to teach in this program, clinical preceptors welcome the opportunity to work with such motivated students and employers are anxious to hire the second degree graduates. If you fit this description, then a second degree program is an option to consider.

In addition to a second bachelor's, there are several other program options for a non-nursing baccalaureate graduate:

1. A generic Master's degree, which is a graduate generalist degree such as Clinical Nurse Leader (CNL). CNL programs range anywhere from 1 to 2 years long, providing advanced education for the nurse at the bedside.
2. A direct entry program for a specialty Master's degree such as a nurse practitioner, clinical nurse specialist, or nurse midwife.
3. An advanced practice degree, DNP.
4. Or a fast-track to a PhD degree in nursing research.

Direct Entry Graduate Degree

If your first baccalaureate degree was not in nursing, you may want to consider going directly into a Master's degree program. The direct entry programs begin with a year of foundation courses in basic nursing, and the support courses of pharmacology, nutrition, and biology. There are the nursing courses plus clinical experience. The second and third year are graduate clinical specialty courses, theory, and research. Take a look at Linda Pellico's wonderful article about nursing as a second career: http://www.nursingcenter.com/CareerCenter/articles.asp: "We'll Leave the Light On for You: There's No Proscribed Path to becoming a Nurse"

There are many paths that lead to nursing. Table 2-2 is a summary of the possibilities.

The *American Journal of Nursing* has several informative articles on a nursing career path in the 2006 Career Guide issue that are accessible online, and they are well worth reading (see http://www.nursingcenter. com/CareerCenter/articles.asp: including "My Big, Fat, Fruitful Nursing Career: Equal Doses of Mind and Spirit." "My Zigzag Career: From Bedside to Pharmaceuticals and Always Looking Ahead," and "The Many Hats of Nursing: What's a Nurse without Patients?"

Table 2-2. Program options to prepare you to be a nurse

Type of Program	Length of Program	Location of Program	Degree Granted	Information
Diploma	3 years	Hospital	Not a college degree unless in collaboration with a community college	Fewer diploma programs, those in the hospital are connected to community colleges
Associate Degree (AD)	2 years	Community College	AD	Many community colleges have nursing programs
Baccalaureate (BS)	4 years	College or University	BS	Traditional 4-year undergraduate degree Many programs are an upper division major with gen. ed. and prerequisite courses the first two years. Nursing courses are junior and senior year
AD to BS	1–2 years	College or University	BS	Many programs for AD grads to earn a BS are online or w/e

(Continued)

Table 2-2. Program options to prepare you to be a nurse (Continued)

Type of Program	Length of Program	Location of Program	Degree Granted	Information
Second Bachelors	15 months-2 years	College or University	BS	A post baccalaureate degree to earn a BS and an RN
Direct-entry MS		College or University	MS	If baccalaureate is not in nursing
BS-MS	5–7 years	College or University	MS	Programs that move right from BS to an MS degree
BS- PhD		College or University	PhD	Fast track to PhD starting with a BS
BS-DNP		College or University	DNP	Start with a BS and go right into a DNP program

CONCLUSION

Nursing programs are demanding, rigorous, and intense. They are also exciting, challenging, and real. Every program from a 2-year Associate's degree to a second Bachelor's degree is designed to prepare you for the role of an RN. There are also many options in nursing. You can work in different specialty areas, different shifts in different locations any where around the world. But to be a nurse takes a special kind of person. How does the nursing role fit for you? The next chapter focuses on a personal assessment.

END-OF-CHAPTER EXERCISE

Envisioning the future can help get you where you want to go. By imagining what area of nursing you'd like to work or the type of facility you can see yourself working in you can begin looking for opportunities that will help you discern if your chosen area is a fit for you. For example, if you are interested in pediatrics, there may be a faculty member conducting research with children with asthma. You could offer to work with the research team. Or there may be a community service opportunity to work with children in the homeless shelter that would provide you with experience. I have had several students interested in ER nursing who became EMTs while they were in college to get a sense of this type of care.

So let's imagine yourself a college graduate and in your first nursing position. Fast-forward 5 years from now:

- How old will you be?

- Where will you be living?

- Where will you be working?

- What do you picture yourself doing as a nurse?

- Can you imagine doing this job everyday?

Okay, now you have a destination in mind. Of course, it is very likely through your classes and clinical experience that this original idea will change. But at least for now, while you are considering nursing, you have a future goal. Your future goal can inspire you to gain experience that will definitely strengthen your school application.

References

American Association of Colleges of Nursing. http://www.aacn.nche.edu.

Beck, C. T., & Gable, R. K. (2003). Postpartum Depression Screening Scale—Spanish version. *Nursing Research, 52*, 296–306.

Beck, C. T., & Gable, R. K. (2001). Further validation of the Postpartum Depression Screening Scale. *Nursing Research, 50*, 155–164.

Beck, C. T. (2001). Predictors of postpartum depression: An update. *Nursing Research, 50*, 275–285.

Self-Assessment

Preparing to Apply to School

Okay, so you are choosing one of the most important professions in health care. Think about it the nurse on the unit for 8- to 12-hour shifts, is in the best position to give voice to the patient's concerns. By choosing nursing, you are choosing a job that really makes a difference. Sarah, an ER nurse, demonstrates the critical role of the nurse in her narrative "The patient knows,"

I met Mr. R sitting bolt upright in the emergency stretcher. He was breathing fast and his skin was this mottled shade of pale, like oatmeal that had been left to sit on the counter. I wondered why the EMTs hadn't called the paramedics for a man who was so obviously sick. He had a nasal cannula in his nose, delivering him his life-giving oxygen. It wasn't enough. He had a terminal condition: pulmonary fibrosis in which the scar tissue on his lungs was depriving his body of oxygen. I changed his oxygen to a high flow nonrebreather mask. After several moments, his color started to improve, a little flush of pink in his otherwise pale cheeks. His oxygen level wave on the monitor now made satisfying hills and valleys, up and down with the rhythm of his heart. The reading was improving: 91%.

I started to step away from him, to start his intravenous and continue my assessment. "I'm going to die," he said as he reached for my hand. I couldn't have pulled away from him if I had wanted. His eyes were locked on mine, with an intensity and calmness. He didn't seem scared, or angry about his fate. His voice was steady and matter-of-fact. It seemed he could have been talking about anything, the weather or something he had seen on TV. Surprisingly, he had a voice. He talked in short, but audible sentences. His breathing was rapid, but he did not seem troubled by it. I asked him why he felt that way, was he in pain? Was his breathing feeling worse? Was there something I could do to make him more comfortable?

"No. I'm just not going to make it."

His statement still caught me off guard. His eyes were closed, so I touched his hand for a moment and then continued at his bedside with starting his IV, drawing blood and hanging normal saline. During this time the doctor came in to see Mr. R. It was a brief encounter; long enough for the doctor to ask him how he was feeling, flip through my notes, do a quick physical assessment, and tell Mr. R that he would need to be admitted. In less than 5 minutes the doctor was off to assess the next patient.

Mr. R was still sitting upright, so I lowered his head slightly in order for him to find a more comfortable position. Emergency stretchers are as comfortable as sunbathing naked on a pile of rocks. He appeared lonely, to want to talk. His eyes searched my face, seemingly saying, "You are going to go now, too?" imploring me to stay. So I stayed with him another moment and asked him about his family. Was he married? Did he have children nearby? His wife of 51 years had died last year of renal failure, but yes, he had a son who was on his way, and four grandchildren. He had pictures in his wallet. They were beautiful, tousled haired young adults with mischievous smiles. He was animated when he spoke of them, his eyes twinkling, regardless of his ragged breaths. I wanted to be able to extend that moment for him, to share in his joy of them, to stay with him and keep him company.

My other patients drew me away; I could hear the ring of a call bell, the shrill and incessant beep of a pump waiting to be checked and there were doctor's orders at hand. He was stabilized and I had other patients who needed me. The emergency department buzzes like a hive, the worker bees never staying in one place too long. While waiting for his orders, I stopped in to see him on my way to another patient's room. When he was finally transferred upstairs to the ICU he looked like a different man from when he had arrived. The cannula was back in place and his oxygen level was maintaining: now 93%. I told him that he looked better. He smiled and said, "I feel just fine." He didn't spend his last moments with me, but he knew better than I did what was before him. Later that night, when I heard the overhead announcement "Code Blue to Critical Care." I knew that it was Mr. R and that he had been right.

Sarah knew how to attend to Mr. R's response to his illness with a thorough physical assessment, titrating his oxygen, and starting his IV. She also knew when to stay and listen, when to be present, and what to notice. You can hear how Sarah worked with Mr. R not only to meet his physical needs but also to have a very difficult conversation. Sarah, the human side of health care, was there when Mr. R needed a nurse.

The nurse plays a central role in taking care of patients. If that is where you picture yourself, on the frontline, then let's start preparing a successful application. Let's start by assessing what characteristics are important for a nurse to have and how that fits with what you bring to nursing.

Reflection 1

Start with what you know from what you have read in Chapters 1 and 2 and what your own experience with health care has taught you.

1. Free-write for 3 minutes essential characteristics of a nurse. Free-writing is when you write what is on your mind for a limited amount of time. So write what comes to mind when you think about what it takes to be a nurse.

2. Set a timer to write for 3 minutes.

3. Start by putting the pen to a blank piece of paper and trying to fill up the page.

4. Even if you start out writing, "I don't know nursing characteristics," just keep writing and you will have the characteristics by the end of your 3 minutes. Promise.

Characteristics of a nurse, free-write for 3 minutes:

Now, from your free-write, make a list of the characteristics you have identified as essential to being a nurse. This is great material for your essay once you have your own ideas down, to hear from others about characteristics of nurses, you may want to Google, "What is a nurse?" or survey the American Association for Nurses web site (http://www.nursingworld.org) or the American Colleges of Nursing web site (http://www.aacn.nche.edu). Keep the list you made in mind, though. We'll come back to it later after you write a little more about yourself. Let's take a look at what you bring to nursing by conducting a Personal Inventory. We all have unique, distinctive, and special characteristics. We know in nursing we need as many kinds of nurses as there are patients. What makes you fit with nursing and what makes you different from other applicants?

PERSONAL INVENTORY

Make a list of what makes you unique, special, distinctive, impressive, or different from any other applicant? This is not the time to be shy.

A. To get started, think about how your friends would describe you.
 1. What friend are you thinking of?
 2. What words would they use to describe you to someone who has not met you yet?
 3. Think of one more friend, maybe from a different aspect of your life. What person are you thinking of?
 4. What words would they use to describe you?
B. Now consider:
 • What is unique about me?
 • What is special or distinctive about me?
 • What is impressive about me?
 • What can I guess would differentiate me from other applicants?

By being honest with yourself, you are already gathering important information for your application to nursing school. This is a time to speak up for yourself. Your goal is for others to get to know you from reading the words you write. Keep going . . .

C. What are your intellectual influences? What writers, books, professors, adults, teachers, coaches have shaped you?

- Who has influenced you? This list can include relatives, friends, teachers, coaches . . .
- What about this person (s) who influenced you, impresses you?
- Make a list of several influences from people to books to situations (jobs, travel) :
  1.
  2.
  3.
  4.

D. How has your high school academic experience prepared you for college? Cite a few particular experiences from high school that come to mind:

E. What are two or three academic accomplishments that have most prepared you for college?
  1.
  2.
  3.

F. Are there any gaps in your academic record that you should explain? Did your grades go up or down one semester?

G. Have you had to overcome unusual hardships (economic, familial, or physical?) in your life?

- What hardship?
- How did you mange this difficult situation?
- And how has this prepared you for managing future difficult situations?

H. What skills do you possess (leadership, communication, social)?

I. Can you tell a story that exemplifies your skills? For example, identify a situation in which you were a leader, a good communicator, or a good friend.

J. What non-academic experiences contribute to your choosing nursing?

- Family/friends?
- Work?
- Volunteering?

K. What have you learned about nursing that has reinforced your interest and conviction that this career decision is right for you? Were there
particular stories in Chapters 1 and 2 that stood out for you? What
was it about the story appealed to you? This is very important to identify, to understand more how you fit and where you fit in nursing.

L. Now that you have reflected on what you bring to nursing, let's go
back to the beginning. Consider what you have read and what you
have listed as essential characteristics of the nurse. How will your
own personal characteristics help you be successful in nursing?

In thinking about coaching you in developing your application, I considered both my own experience and what students have to say. A common theme of my experience and the results of the student survey indicate
that the characteristics that you need to apply to nursing school are the
same characteristics that you will need to succeed as a nursing student as
well the same characteristics you will need to perform as a nursing professional. In other words, the motivation, drive, organization, and forethought
that you need to prepare a school application are the same characteristics
that you will need to be a nursing student. So you can start developing
your nursing potential right here, right now, during the application
process.

The four themes for developing a successful application are:

1. Organization: plan
2. Connection: develop key relationships
3. Curiosity: ask questions
4. Assertiveness: speak up

In nursing practice, we look for new nurses who can organize their
work and prioritize their responsibilities. We know from research that the
type of relationships nurses have with their patients, the positive professional relationships nurses have with physicians, and the collegial connections nurses have with other nurses empower nurses to provide the best
patient care. Empowering nurse-patient-physician relationships enables the
nurse to develo p expertise (Roche, 2004). Not all nurses become experts.
But if you have the right working relationships you have a good chance of
going all the way from the beginning novice to the top expert. Experts
know how to think critically. Developing your curiosity is the initial step for
critical thinking. But nothing works, not organizing, not relationships nor
curiosity, if you do not let others know your opinion by being assertive and

speaking up! In the application process, these four essential career characteristics will assist you in preparing a successful application, beginning with organization.

BE ORGANIZED

Nursing education takes time, commitment, and money. The application process alone will take your time, emotional investment, and financial support. To make good use of your time and money, start by being organized.

- If you are a **junior** in high school, you have time to take the requirements and electives that will help your application. Think about making yourself stand out among the hundreds of applicants. Okay, don't think about the 100s, that's too scary, just think about you and how to enhance your profile with good grades, extracurricular activities, and community service.

- If you are a **senior**, you still have time to study to keep that Grade Point Average (GPA) up and choose an elective that would enhance your application. Our local high school offers an elective course on death and dying and another elective on the Holocaust. Both of these courses would be good electives for future nurses.

- If you are a **transfer** student, concentrate on studying to get good grades. Get to know your professor or teaching assistant so they can guide you in studying and know who you are in the class. A teacher or teaching assistant is ideal for writing a letter of recommendation. Your prenursing requirements predict how well you will do with nursing courses, so you will want to demonstrate to the admissions committee that you can handle college-level courses—in fact, that you can do well in them!

- If you are a **second Bachelor's** student, consider how to frame your education and your past experience to focus on what you have learned that connects with what you know about nursing. Get to know the professors teaching the prerequisite courses so they can write you a recommendation. Look for educational, community, and leadership opportunities to enhance your application.

- If you are **starting later** in life, I say, "Come on in!" For your application, organize your life experience so you can demonstrate your motivation and fit with nursing.

Let's look at a typical application and see what nursing schools are looking for. You can plan ahead by going to any school's web site and find their specific application online. You can also download the Common Undergraduate Application as a PDF document from the following web site: http://app.commonapp.org/.

In addition, you can obtain application forms for community college programs, second Bachelor's degree programs, and RN-BS programs from the following web sites:

Community college application example: http://www.gcc.mass.edu/admission/application.html

Second Bachelor's application example:

http://www.umass.edu/nursing/programs/pro_ug_second_bach/ug_secondary.html

RN-BS application example:

http://www.umass.edu/nursing/programs/pro_ug_RN_to_BS/ug_rnbs.html

As you can see from the application forms, colleges are looking at:

- Your high school GPA and your college GPA
- The types and level of courses you took
- Your extracurricular activities
- Community activities
- Work history
- Leadership activities in
    - Arts
    - Sports
    - Academics
    - Community service

Whew! Even writing that list is intimidating! So let's break the application down into manageable steps and take each step one at a time, beginning with your GPA.

GPA and Coursework

You and I both know that the "authorities" believe that your GPA indicates how well you've performed in school. We also know that your GPA is a fraction of who you really are but it's a beginning piece of information for an Admissions Committee to consider. Now, every college wants you to do well. So, the college is looking for applicants who have a track record of doing well in school. Make sense? Let's look at your GPA and the grades that you received in high school or any college courses:

High school GPA:_____

High school courses:	Course	Grade
	_____	_____
	_____	_____
	_____	_____
	_____	_____
	_____	_____
	_____	_____
	_____	_____
	_____	_____

College GPA:_____

Reflection 2

Let's build on what you've done well. The following questions will help you reflect on what works for you and this will help you be able to talk yourself in the essay and the interview. Think about:

1. What courses have you done well in?

2. Why do you think you did well that course?
   a. Was it the teacher? Who was the teacher?
   b. List a few teacher characteristics that help you learn.
   c. Was it the content of the course? What turned you on about this content?
   d. What class activities worked for you? Recall what you did in class or for homework that assisted you in learning the content.

Reflection 3

1. What previous courses did you do well in?

2. Do you know what it was about the coursework that prevented you from doing well?

3. Is it worth considering improving this grade? How?

With these answers, you are beginning to describe yourself as a learner. This will assist you not only in presenting yourself in an application and knowing yourself as a learner, but also it will be a good preparation for an interview. In addition, when you know more about your learning style, you can anticipate your learning needs in your future nursing program. Who are you as a learner?

Howard Gardner talks about the eight intelligences (http://www.pz. harvard.edu). Think about yourself and the intelligences that are your strength. The first two, linguistic and logical-mathematical intelligence, are primarily IQ; the six other intelligences are additional ways of viewing the world.

1. **Linguistic intelligence** includes being able to articulate your thoughts in spoken and written language and the ability to learn new languages, and the capacity to use language to accomplish certain goals. A strong vocabulary and the ability to express yourself verbally, and in writing all add up to linguistic intelligence.

2. **Logical-mathematical intelligence** involves the capacity to analyze problems, formulate mathematical operations, and investigate issues in scientific manner. This intelligence not only involves numbers but also the ability to detect patterns, reason deductively, and think logically. Problem solving, decision making, and planning are related to logical intelligence.

3. **Musical intelligence** includes skill in the performance, composition, and appreciation of musical patterns. Playing an instrument, singing, or having rhythm is musical intelligence.

4. **Bodily-kinesthetic intelligence** is the potential of using one's whole body or parts of the body to coordinate bodily movements. There are many types of body intelligence such as dancing, sports, or rock climbing.

5. **Spatial intelligence** involves thinking in picture and images. Some people have this ability to conjure up a space, like painters, architects, or city planners.

6. **Interpersonal intelligence** is concerned with the capacity to understand the intentions, motivations, and desires of other people, often referred to as emotional intelligence. Emotional intelligence includes:

   a. Self-awareness of strengths and weaknesses

   b. Self-management, meaning the ability to manage emotions in different situations

   c. Social awareness, which is understanding the perspective of others

   d. Social skill indicates the ability to create comfortable relationships in which interactions leave each individual feeling heard, recognized, and connected.

7. **Intrapersonal intelligence** means the capacity to understand oneself, to appreciate one's feelings, fears, and motivations. Intrapersonal intelligence is similar to self-awareness.

8. **Naturalist intelligence** enables human beings to recognize and draw on certain features of the natural world, feeling comfortable in nature and drawing strength from natural surroundings.

Each intelligence provides you with an opportunity to describe yourself, assess where you need support and build on what you do well.

Before you fill out the application and before any interview, you will need to think about what supports your learning and what inhibits your learning. Demonstrating the ability to be reflective is an essential nursing skill. Reflection meaning you can look back on a situation and learn from it. For example, nurses talk about reflecting back on their shift on their drive home, reviewing whether they did everything possible for their patient, if they called the pharmacy or if they sent the tests to the lab. You can practice reflection by looking back on your own school experience and identify what you learned from the positive and not so positive experiences.

Reflection 4

1. What positive school experience comes to mind? What did you learn from this experience?

2. Think of a difficult school experience. What did you learn from that experience?

Keep these responses in mind for your essay.

Extracurricular Activities, Community Service, and Leadership

Now some high school students are natural school participants; they join everything, they feel they have something to contribute and enjoy extracurricular activities. Other students are into their own thing, sports, theater, or community service. In any of these areas you can build your learning and leadership potential. Many students, by contrast, think it is dorky to look interested in school or community activities. I was one of those "too cool for school" kids:

At the end of my sophomore year my parents transferred me to a new, out of town high school. Just understanding the classes, doing the homework, and making new friends was enough for me. All the club and sport people were not part of my new crowd anyways. But I did volunteer at the local hospital pediatric unit during the summer. I loved taking care of babies and kids. Community activities worked better for me than in-school participation.

The problem with the too-cool-for-school view is that colleges want you to be involved in their college life too, so they are looking for high school students with a track record of being a member of something. And guess what? When you graduate from college, hospitals are looking for college students that have demonstrated active involvement in college life. I wish somebody had told me this. Think about what works for you. If your goal is to get into nursing, choose something in school or in the community you can be involved in that is related to health care and maybe even consider a leadership position.

Reflection 5

1. What interests you in your school? Art, science, sports?

2. What interests you in the community? Volunteering at the shelter, working with the elderly?

3. Is it possible to volunteer at a hospital?

4. Several schools actually require applicants to work as nursing assistant. Being a Certified Nursing Assistant (CNA) requires a training course that costs anywhere from $300 to $500. However, some nursing homes offer the course for free when you commit to work there. Consider this opportunity.

5. Are you a non-joiner? Then what can you do to demonstrate you want to help others?

Once you have described your interests, consider your leadership abilities, we all have them, some just show up sooner than others. Read on . . .

Leadership

Okay, so now you volunteer for the yearbook and serve meals at the homeless shelter. This is good, very good. Picture this:

- When you are in a yearbook meeting or at the shelter, they ask: who can be in charge of the budget?
- Who can chair the committee on sports in the yearbook?
- OR, who can chair the committee on nutrition at the community shelter?

Put your hand up.

Not that you have to volunteer for just anything, but join in when something interests you. Chairing committees is a learned skill. I teach college students about the skills of group dynamics and I am still learning how to chair a meeting effectively myself. The job of facilitating a committee changes depending on the people you are working with and the task you need to accomplish. Leadership is something you learn.

When I was in college, I ran for the position of senator in the student government. Senator, some people naturally gravitate toward these titles and that's great but class senator, that was so not me, except, I had a college rule I wanted to change and I was bound and determined to do so. Back in the day, we were not allowed to wear jeans to class. I know, it was a long time ago and even then I thought it was ridiculous. I looked into how students can change college rules and learned that the student voice is listened to through the student government. So I went for it. Now the moral of the story is just don't volunteer for anything but find something you are genuinely interested in, even if it is just jeans. Hey, I got to be senator and got to wear jeans and moved on from there. It was a humble start. You can start, too.

You can begin learning leadership skills by volunteering and then learning on the job. Start by choosing something that is of interest to you, arts, sports, science, nature, poetry, photography, etc. Every one of your interests will vastly improve your application to nursing school or any school for that matter. Look back at that application. See how they ask for community service and leadership positions? You want to be able to fill something in that blank. You will also need to write something in your college essay about leadership. Why not start developing those skills now?

What is leadership anyway? Good question. One look at the management section in any bookstore will tell you that a lot of experts are trying to answer the leadership question. Actually we all know someone we would consider a leader. Think about this.

Reflection 6

1. Name an individual you would consider a leader.

2. What makes you think of this person as a leader?

3. What do they do that means leadership?
   a.
   b.
   c.
   d.

Each of us can develop our leadership capability by understanding what leadership skills are. Leadership doesn't necessarily mean you are in an official leadership position. In fact, I am sure that you can name friends that have leadership abilities but are not in charge. You can have leadership skills without an official title. As a nursing student, you will be expected to take the lead with your patient by confronting problems, speaking up for your patient, or in coordinating discharge plans. Each nurse is expected to have leadership capability. I am sure that you named some of the following five leadership skills in your own list. I am also sure you have some of these leadership skills. These five skills are what experts (Kouzes & Posner, 1989, http://www.leadershipchallenge.com) describe as leadership skills:

1. **Challenge the status quo**: Leaders question, wonder, think of new ways of doing things.

2. **Inspire a shared vision**: Leaders have a dream of what could be, a desire to create something new, to change how things are, and bring others on board.

3. **Enable others to act**: No leader acts on their own, whether they are leaders for the good or leaders that create bad situations they are always working with a team. Leaders know how to build teams get support from others and encourage collaboration so everyone works together.

4. **Model the way**: Leaders model what they want. As Gandhi said, become the change you want. Then leaders create detailed plans so others can join in. Whether it is a script for a play or a game plan, people need to know where they are going and how to get there before they will agree to join you.

5. **Encourage the heart**: People need support along the way when working on a project or playing a sport. They need encouragement, positive feedback, helpful advice, recognition for their good work, and rewards that have meaning. You know this. You know how good it feels to be encouraged and recognized.

Think about times in your life when you have used one of these skills.

Reflection 7

Think of a time when you have put at least one of the leadership skills to use. I know you have challenged the status quo with your parents. When else have you used one, two, or three of these leadership skills?

1.

2.

3.

Okay, that is a good beginning. Keep these leadership skills in front of you. I know you will think of other examples.

Can you see how to use an example of leadership skills in your application essay? Keep the five skills in mind for when we get to the essay. In this narrative, here is how a staff nurse, Rachel, takes the lead in attending to her patient's wishes:

I was caring for an older patient who was newly diagnosed with cancer; she was at a point where she was unable to eat through her mouth. A feeding tube was the only option to keep this woman alive. The patient's daughter was strongly involved in her mother's care and would do anything to keep her mother alive. This morning the physician ordered a feeding tube to be placed. I went in to explain the situation to my patient since the physicians had not been in to see her yet. The patient, being alert and oriented, refused the feeding tube. The physician's response was, "The patient has no choice. She needs the tube and the daughter wants her to have the tube as well and the daughter is the health care proxy. The patient will have the tube placed." As an advocate for my patient I was going to do anything to follow my patient's wishes. I was now in an ethical dilemma. My feelings at this time were for my patient. I knew I had to be my patient's voice, so I decided to go higher and went to the ethics committee to review the situation with them. The committee agreed that the patient was alert and oriented and was fully capable of making her own decisions; therefore she would not have the feeding tube. I, as a nurse, have to stick to what my patient's wishes and needs are. In this case, I personally did not agree with my patient's decision. I thought she had good quality of life according to my standards, but for her she did not feel this way and I respected her thoughts and fought for her rights as my patient.

Rachel assumed a leadership role in caring for her patient. Rachel was there when her patient needed her and consulted with experts on the ethics committee when she needed to take it further. Taking the lead is a key role for any nurse. You will want to demonstrate that you have leadership potential in your application.

When writing your application, it is helpful to have a goal or destination in mind so you can stay focused on why you are doing all of this work. Let's think about your goal for your future.

Reflection 8: How to get from here to there?

When we start off to a place we have not been before, whether it is a place or a goal, the best approach is to first know where you are going and second, have a set of directions and a map on how to get there. Of course, sometimes we don't have either directions or map, I've tried this many times and I must admit going to the unknown without a map does not work that well. So let's at least start with a destination and then work to formulate your map. Start with 6 years from now, If you have a goal out in front of you it will help you move toward the future by:

- Knowing what courses to choose
- Knowing what activities to be involved in
- Knowing what topics to read about
- Knowing what people to meet

If you envision 6 years from now being an emergency room nurse then right now you want to pay attention to information about emergency nursing. You may want to take an EMT course or pay attention to current topics in the news about emergency care. For instance, there is a recent Institute of Medicine (IOM, http://www.iom.edu) report that has been in the news: emergency rooms are in crisis because of overcrowding and too few hospital beds. Think about how knowledgeable you'd look if you were asked what kind of nurse you wanted to be and then said you were concerned about the recent news about the conditions in the ER. Whoa, impressive! So consider your destination:

- What sort of nurse do you envision yourself being?
- Are you dressed in scrubs from head to toe, gowned, masked, and gloved for the operating room?
- Are you dashing around the ER?
- Are you feeding a tiny baby, a 46-year-old patient with cancer, or a 92-year-old struggling with dementia?
- Are you in the hospital, in a home, or working for hospice caring for the dying?
- Can you see yourself working with individuals in a psychiatric unit?
- Do you see yourself as a nurse scientist? Or a nursing professor?
- Where do you see yourself as a nurse? In the hospital, in a clinic, in a neighborhood?

Visit web sites to get some ideas. Here is an e-mail a student sent me that is focused on Massachusetts, but you can find these in any state, Jill recommends:

As early as possible beginning nursing students should navigate and get to know that many opportunities are out there. Students can e-mail the hospital's Human Resources department or visit human resources in person at a hospital where they would like to shadow a nurse. Many hospitals have programs to show high school students nursing options. Here are some great sites that I visit regularly:

http://www.mhalink.org/public/mahospitals/

http://www.nln.org/CLWebsites/MARI/about.htm

MA/RI League for Nursing provides scholarships for juniors in nursing school and also for RNs.

http://www.nursema.org/

http://www.massnurses.org/

www.nursingworld.org

Write down the nurse you want to be 6 years from now.
Okay, good, now we have a destination.
That vision of your future role as a nurse will most likely change, but for now you need something that will pull you forward, something you can get excited about, something that will assist you in filling out applications. Connecting to the right people will also assist in the application process.

CREATE RELATIONSHIPS

In developing your application, you can begin by thinking about what new connections would inform you about nursing. You may need to reach out beyond the people you know to connect with professional nurses. *The more informed you are about applying to school and the requirements of school, the better position you will be in.*

Okay, so let's connect with people who can give us the information you need.

Reflection 9

Think about it. Who do you need to talk with to learn about nursing school? Off the top of your head, make a list of people that can help you in this process of applying to school:

1.

2.

3.

4.

5.

Do you know a nurse, or does your mom or dad? That would be a place to start. Many hospitals have programs where they bring high school students in to observe. One way to prepare for the future is to see if there is a club in your school for future careers. Check it out.

Consider volunteering to get some firsthand experience. When you volunteer in a nursing home (they will welcome you) or a hospital, get to know a nurse or two so they could write you a letter of recommendation. Letters from professional nurses will get you further than letters from family friends, *so you need to meet some nurses.*

What about all those school and extracurricular activities that you are involved in? Review the requirements for the letters of recommendation in the school application. Admissions committees want to hear about leadership, critical thinking, and your relationship building, so someone other than your mom and dad have to know you well enough so that they can write a letter honestly speaking to qualities that suit you for nursing school, such as responsibility, dependability, and motivation. These attributes do not have to be connected to health care. For instance, you could have demonstrated responsibility when you worked on a project in school or in your community. Curiosity is another trait that is valued in nursing.

BE CURIOUS

If you are in **high school,** ask your guidance counselor questions about a nursing career. Visit the school nurse and ask about her career path. If you are in **college,** transferring into nursing, get to know the people in the nursing school, the secretary (they know everything!) the junior students, the senior students, the faculty.

Megan, a nursing student writes:

Learn how to deal with the school of nursing administration. They can help and hurt you. Be aggressive. Ask questions. Do not be intimidated by them, even if they seem annoyed. Being silent gets you nowhere. Get to know your advisor and make yourself known.

These are words directly from a junior student. If you are a prenursing student, ask questions in class, meet with the teaching assistant, and take advantage of any extra study support that the professor offers. Younger students often withhold from asking questions so they will not look stupid. Take a lesson from the **second Bachelor's** students. These students have already graduated with a BS degree and sometimes have a Master's degree when they decide to make a change in their career and come back to school to become a nurse. The second Bachelor's students are excellent students. I have not heard a professor say otherwise. Part of the reason that the faculty think so highly of the second Bachelor's student is because they come prepared to class, they are motivated to learn, and they ask questions, lots of questions. All the time. In every class. Follow their lead, come forward, and ask questions.

When I asked a group of second Bachelor's students what they wish they knew before they came into the program, they told me:

- You are in charge of your education: be proactive.
- Don't be afraid to ask lots of questions
- Forgive yourself for not knowing everything

I told you that they have wisdom to offer the rest of us! The second Bachelor's students are experienced in academic settings. They know it is essential to be an assertive student.

BE ASSERTIVE

The nursing profession is over 100 years old. Professional nursing was started by an upstart, who went against her parent's wishes, was a statistical expert, a revered researcher, and went to the front lines of a war to nurse the wounded. She was intelligent, outspoken, and influential. She was Florence Nightingale, the founder of modern nursing. Although we started with a dynamic leader, many still envision nurses as subservient, silent angels of mercy. That is not the case. To practice safe nursing, nurses must be vocal.

With over 100,000 medical errors a year, when one in five medications being given are incorrect, nurses are in a position to make a difference. Nurses are on the sharp end of care, meaning they stand between the treatment prescribed and the treatment given. The nurse decides when to call a physician in so she must know what is going on with the patient. The nurse reads the physician's orders and decide where they fit with this patient, is this the right medication, the right dosage? Is the patient allergic to this medication? The nurse sees the patients' response to treatments, the patient's response to surgery, and the patient's response to their illness. Nurses must speak up to manage and to coordinate patient care. Sarah recognizes that her role is to speak up and advocate for her patient:

I was taking care of this particular patient named "Joe." Joe was a very sick man. His kidneys were shutting down, he had metastatic cancer. When he first arrived on the floor, Joe was very aware of his surroundings. He knew exactly what he wanted to do. He wanted to die. However, the doctor in charge of his renal issues had other things in mind for Joe. He wanted Joe to start dialysis and convinced Joe's son that this was the best thing to do. I would sit in the room with Joe, and he would talk only about dying. As the days went by, Joe did become more and more confused. He started on dialysis as the son wanted and Joe got madder and madder. At times Joe was so angry that we had to use two-point wrist restraints and sometimes four-point wrist and ankle restrains. After seeing this for 2 months, I went to my Nursing Manager and explained the situation to her. She agreed with me that this was an ethical/advocacy issue. The ethics committee was called and the doctor was contacted to get the plan of care from him. Shortly after, dialysis was stopped, we no longer had to restrain Joe, and he was put on comfort measures only.

Nurses speak for the patient, advocate for patients, and prevent medical errors by using their voice. You can start developing your voice even before you enter nursing so that you will be ready to assume the role when you enter the program.

Reflection 10

Think of a time you stood up for somebody.

1. Who did you stand up for?

2. What was the situation?

You have experience being an advocate, learn how to articulate that experience.

Standing up for someone else is advocating for them. Nurses are patient's advocates. From the story you wrote above you know how to advocate for someone else. Now it is time to advocate for yourself.

CONCLUSION

Developing a strong nursing school application takes time, investment, and motivation. To do your best you must be organized, develop key relationships, be curious, and be assertive. All of these traits will help you in designing your own, unique application and they will also lay the groundwork for being a successful nursing student.

END-OF-CHAPTER EXERCISE: LETTER OF RECOMMENDATION

Letters of recommendation are important testimony to your character, if the letters are done well. A letter is written well if it addresses the interests of the school and the assets of the applicant. The creative aspect of writing a letter is to have the school's interests and the applicant's assets match. Often we inadvertently request letters of recommendation from individuals who are unaware of what the school is looking for. When you request a letter, it is helpful to inform the person about the particular school you are applying to and about your own recent interests and accomplishments. For example, one school's mission may have an emphasis on diversity and another school may focus on global health. How can your letter writers speak about the school's focus?

As you can see, there is more that goes into letter-writing than just asking a friend to recommend you for nursing school. You have to help the person know what needs to be said. So, let's practice by writing a letter of recommendation for yourself. Seriously, this is the best approach to understanding the information needed to write a good letter.

1. Choose a nursing school on the Web

2. Read the school's mission statement. That will tell you the program's focus.

3. Read the application carefully to see if an essay is required and what the focus of the essay should be. Knowing about the focus of the essay will give you more information about the school's interests.

4. Find out if the school asks for the letter of recommendation to address specific points, such as, motivation, leadership, or intellectual abilities.

5. Find out if the school requires letters from a person in health care, education, or employers. Many schools are very specific in their request for letters of recommendation.

Now write a letter that talks about your assets and the school's interests. This will help you be more specific when you ask others to write letters for you so you will get just the letter you need!

___

References

Gardner, H. (1983, 1993). *Frames of mind: The theory of multiple intelligences.* New York: Basic Books.

Kouzes, J., & Posner, B. (2003). *The leadership challenge* (3rd ed.). Jossey Bass.

Roche, J. (2004). *Work empowerment, work relationships and expertise in experienced acute care nurses.* Unpublished dissertation, University of Massachusetts, Amherst, MA.

[CHAPTER 4]

On the Right Track
Applications, Essays, and Interviews

Finally! Time to fill out the application. Now that you have some ideas about the type of program you'd like to apply to, let's fill out an application. This is a big step. Completing the application and essay will take your time, a personal commitment and an investment of energy. The good news is, because you have responded to all the reflective exercises in Chapter 3, you already have what is required for any application form. Plus, you have already identified your unique abilities, your special interests, and your leadership capabilities, so you are more than halfway through the essay. Still, give yourself plenty of time to fill out applications. All good writing takes several drafts.

You want the Admissions Committee to take your application very seriously, to read every detail, to note your volunteer work, to nod their heads in recognition when they read about your leadership abilities. You want each faculty member on the Admission Committee to weigh your strengths favorably in comparison to all the other applicants. Am I right? Okay, so if you want the Admissions Committee to do all of that work then you need to put the work into the application process so it is in great shape when it goes out the door. You need to let the Admissions Committee know who you are through the schools you have attended, coursework you have completed, and extracurricular activities that you have been involved in. You want to create a unique, insightful essay that reads like a story; a story that each individual on the Admissions Committee will remember. You'll want to have the right professional letters of recommendation that can describe the characteristics you have that are important in nursing so that the committee can see you are a good match for their profession. Once you have actively responded (which means that you actually wrote the answers out) to the questions in Chapter 3, you are way ahead of the candidate who just plunges into the application packet.

Filling in the answers to the questions asked in applications is not an easy task, not because the answers are so difficult but because we have been raised not to boast and not to be selfish. Yet, that attitude of holding back may prevent us from letting others know who we are. Think of the application as an opportunity to share information. This is a time when you are trying to have a room full of strangers judge you, so you want to give them ample evidence to choose you for the nursing program.

Some schools don't require an essay; others require two or three essays and an interview! Try to think of the more opportunities to interact with the school; through essays or interviews, you'll have more opportunities to convince the school that you are the right person for the job. Let's start with the essay, rehearse the interview, and request the recommendations.

THE ESSAY

The essay offers you the opportunity to present yourself in your own words in your own style. The essay will give the committee the opportunity to look beyond the numbers of grades and test scores and into a narrative about you. The essay not only tells the Admissions Committee more about you but also the essay demonstrates how you think, how you organize your thoughts, and how you present yourself. This means that you have control over the style and content of your essay, so be thoughtful about what you want the Admissions Committee to read. To create a winning essay, you will need to:

1. Carefully read the directions for the essay
2. Review the school web site
3. Be original and creative:
   a. Mind map
   b. Free write

Directions

The first step to writing the essay is to read the directions *slowly* and *carefully*. Ask yourself, what is the focus of the essay? For example, one school asks about diversity:

"Diversity is a core value of our school and a necessary value of nursing. Respect and dignity are critical to understanding diversity. Describe a situation when one or more of these values was challenged for you and describe your response."

Another school requests that the essay focus on leadership:

"Leadership is a core behavior of our graduates. Describe your leadership capabilities, decisions you made, and your ability to work on a team."

Some baccalaureate programs at large universities review the essay from the general application. The general application essay may be:

"Daily life presents us with choices, some more challenging than others. What significant choices have you made and discuss the consequences of your actions. What was the impact of these decisions on your life?"

"What does the phrase "community of learners" mean to you? How would your background and experience help contribute to our community of learners?"

"Our place in the world is influenced by significant others and significant events. Describe a person or event that has had a profound impact on your view of the world."

"In 500 words or less, describe any positive or negative personal circumstances or academic experiences that you feel are important for us to know about."

Or

"Why do you want to be a nurse?"

You can see, just from this small sample of essay directions, the different types of essays that large universities and small colleges request. There is no such thing as one essay fits all. Some schools actually ask for essays on three topics! So you will need to give yourself ample time to create your response and then critique your writing.

Web Site

Now that you know the essay focus, before you even pick up your pen or pull up "new blank document," you'll need to look over the school's web site. A school web page is where you go to check out what the program is all about, how the program is described and to get a sense of the school. You look at a school web site to see what the program feels like, is the information hard to find? or is it accessible and easy to follow? But, just as face book, you cannot tell everything but you can get a feeling for the school and its programs.

Reflection 1

1. When you first open a school Web page, what do you see?

2. Is the image pleasing to you?

3. How would you describe the greeting you get from the homepage? Official? Friendly? Inviting? Cold?

4. Can you negotiate the site easily?

5. When was the site last updated?

Of course, keep in mind the old saying, "You can't tell a book by its cover." Same goes for web sites, and for most sites Web designers are creating the image, but, still, we can work to get a sense of what is behind the curtains. Just like the Wizard of Oz, the information on the site will help us to peek into the program.

Reflection 2

For the purposes of the essay, you will want to note the language used on the web site.

1. Does the school web site emphasize Community? Scholarship? Leadership?

2. What is the school's Mission Statement? The mission is a statement reflecting the purpose of the school. Does the mission fit with your purpose of going into nursing?

3. What is the school's philosophy? The philosophy is a statement of the school's values. Do these values fit with your values?

4. What is the school's vision? The vision statement is where the school is heading in the future. Do you see yourself heading in the same direction as this school?

Once you have searched a few different sites with these questions in mind, you will see what I mean; some will be attractive to you, others will not.

- Carefully read the web sites of the nursing schools that you have chosen.

- Write specifically about their program by noting the words that are used on the site:

— Do they talk about critical thinkers? (a current buzz word). Then use critical thinking in your essay.

— Do they talk about advocacy? Teaching? Literacy?

— Locate the buzz words of that specific school. Pull these words out.

— Consider where these words can show up on your application.

Of course, the web site is only the beginning. A visit to the school is what will really tell you a lot about how you feel you fit. Recently, an applicant told me that she should have started with a visit because she could tell so much about the environment, the faculty, and the students. When she visited the campus, she got a much better idea about what would work for her and probably would have sent out fewer applications to places she had no interest in studying. (More on visits later in this chapter.) For now, with the directions for the essay and information from the school web site, let's start writing.

Tap into Creativity

Mind Maps

A strategy used to kick in the creative juices is a mind map, sometimes called clustering. You probably used this technique in high school to develop a topic for a paper. Well, now the topic is you and the mind map can be a useful tool to generate ideas about yourself. To create a mind map, read the following instructions:

1. The first step is to make sure you have your pad and pencil with you.
2. Start a mind map by drawing a big sun in the middle of the page. Try it. BIG sun, you know, circle and rays. Good.
3. Now to start to write this essay put your main focus in the center of the circle. Write out: "diversity in my life" or "my leadership abilities" in the center of the sun.
4. Then, focus on the statement in the center. Focus by centering yourself. Center yourself (which merely means trying to put all the other chatter in your head aside for the moment and be here. Right here). Center yourself by taking 3 deep breaths. Okay, breathe deeply: one, breath, two, breath, three, breath. Are you with me?
5. Now focus on the words in the middle of the circle for a moment or two.

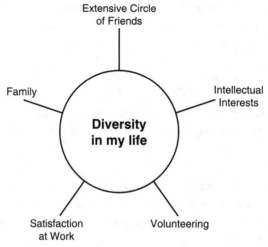

Figure 4-1. Example of a mind map.

6. Next, at the end of each ray write an idea that comes to mind about the statement in the middle.

7. Finally, free-write for 2 minutes, including all of your ideas that are at the end of the rays.

8. You have now engaged the creative side of your brain and begun your essay. Way to go!

You can create a mind map for each aspect of the essay. For example if the essay focus is to be about diversity, then write diversity at the center of the sun and go back to step 3. If the next essay is "why you want to be a nurse" put that statement in the middle of the sun. You get the picture.

Figure 4-1 is an example of a mind map. This picture is worth a thousand words.

Free-Write

Free-writing is another way to jump-start your creative brain. Free-writing can be used with a mind map like we did in the section above or just put the pen to the page and start out writing. Peter Elbow has written the classic books on developing your writing ability. It is not too late to pick one up and learn some very helpful writing strategies. You will use these writing strategies all the way through college and into graduate school. Because many of us are not confident in our writing abilities, it is worth investing in some support. Elbow's *Writing without Teachers, Writing with*

Power, and *Everyone Can Write* are wonderful resources on writing. In his book, *Writing with Power,* Peter describes the process of free-writing. Free-writing begins with an idea:

1. Let's say your idea is "a leadership challenge" or a topic from your mind map that you'd like to develop.
2. Once you have a topic in mind, put the pen to the page and write for at least 10 minutes, up to 20 minutes, in response to your chosen topic. The best way to stay within your time limits is to set a timer for 10 minutes.
3. When you put the pen to the page do not worry about the mechanics of writing or spelling or grammar, just try to fill up the page.
4. Let yourself go where your pen goes; even if it looks like you are off topic, keep going.
5. If you get stuck, keep writing, "I don't know what to write" and keep going.
6. Don't stop until the timer rings. After the 10-minute free-write, you will have many ideas about a challenging leadership experience. Promise.

The next step is to put the free-write aside and come back to it later to see how you can organize your ideas. The next time you pick up your free-write, look for some patterns or themes. What stands out for you? Can the patterns be prioritized and organized into an outline?

Consider doing several different free-writes at different times in the day. Julia Cameron, from her creativity book *The Artist's Way,* suggests doing morning pages by free-writing three pages right as you wake up. Some students say morning writing helps, others prefer writing right before they go to bed. Think of free-writing as building your writing muscle. Just as with any muscle-building plan, you want to stretch out by doing a little writing each day so that you can build up your writing ability. By a little writing, I mean try writing morning pages for 10 minutes a day. You cannot expect yourself to just "write the essay." You need to build that writing muscle, find an area that interests you from the mind map, and free-write to that topic.

The mind map and free-write are designed to kick in the right side of the brain, the creative side. In writing you want to engage the creative side for at least 80% of the time whether the writing is for an essay or for a class assignment. When you write you will want to separate out the creator and the critic. Writers block occurs when the critic and creator are intertwined. You write a word and the critic in your head says, "That's not the right word" or the computer says, "That's not the right spelling." So the critic in you pauses to think of the right word and your creative energy goes out the window. Even just respelling a word invites the critic side of your brain in and the critic will stop the creative juices from flowing. To write your essay you have to set aside the critic so you can be creative. Only in the last 20% of your writing will you get serious with the critic and clean up the organization, make sure that the essay flows well, check grammar, spelling, and punctuation. Because the computer underlines spelling mistakes, some people choose to free-write in long hand on paper before employing the computer. This prewrite is just the first stage of writing, but it is so necessary.

You have probably learned about stages of writing in high school and you thought it was just for your class assignment. Well, guess what? Writing your admission essay is a time you can use all five stages of writing. I know this is getting tedious, going through all this preparation to write an essay, but this is your one chance to be you, to use your voice with this invisible committee, so you'll want to do it well. Keep going. Here is a step-by-step approach to writing:

Stages of Writing

1. Prewriting
2. Drafting
3. Revising
4. Editing/proof reading
5. Final draft

Prewriting (Preparing to Write)

- Free-write in a journal format, use morning pages or bedtime musings.
- Identify the purpose of your essay and the audience you are writing for. Who is going to read this essay? Keep your audience in mind when you write.
- Research, take notes, gather information as you are thinking about your essay.
- Brainstorm with a peer group what you might write about.
- Create a mind map and free-write.

Drafting (Putting Thoughts on Paper)

There will be several drafts of any official paper, so plan on at least three drafts for your essay.

This is your first draft. Build on your free-write or mind map.

- Compose freely, without concern for mechanics right now, you are still in the creative stage.

- Don't be concerned about length, write everything that comes to mind, you can cut back later.

- Create a working thesis statement. A thesis statement goes in the introduction and states the purpose of your essay. This statement can change so we are calling it a working thesis statement for now.

- From your creative writing, pull out three points that you want to make in your essay.

- Write the first sentence, which is called the "hook" because it draws the reader in. The hook could be a question or a provocative statement.

Revising (Taking Another Look)

- Maintain focus on the required content for the essay.

- Put your paragraphs in a logical order.

- Keep your essay fresh and energized by paying attention to detail and language. Think "show," don't just "tell." This is very important guideline for writing: show, don't tell. This means don't just tell the reader, "I am a caring person," but show how you have been caring with a little story. Details help the reader see the picture you are creating. This is your one chance for the Admissions Committee to know you through the details you present.

- The essay is an opportunity for the Committee to evaluate your thinking and writing ability. Of course, you will learn more about thinking and writing in college, but you want to show them you have a good start.

After you have revised for the first time, ask yourself:
  – Are my goals clearly stated?
  – Do I explain why I selected this school in particular?
  – Did I demonstrate knowledge of their program?
  – Have I included interesting details to support my claims about myself?

Share this draft with a peer or two and consider peer-editing your essay. Peer-editing is when you read your essay out loud to an individual or your peer reads your essay on their own. Before you have a friend read your essay, make it clear what you want from the listener. A peer-edit guide should not include too much; maybe you want to hear from your peer:

- What do you like?

- What stays with you?

- Where do you get lost?

- What should I emphasize?

- Reading out loud can be very informative. When you read you can hear how the words flow and you will be able to tell if they are choppy or vague. Don't be shy about this. If you want the Admissions Committee to read your easy, you should read it also.
- Invite discussion from your peer reader.
- Add to, delete from, rearrange, and revise this draft.

Editing/Proofreading

Now we have to get technical here. This is where the critic comes in.

- Read the entire essay aloud to yourself, again.
- Check spelling and grammar, then even go over spell check to see if you have the right words. Sometimes as you are going along a word is inserted from the thesaurus that does not say what you had in mind.
- Do you have an introduction, body, and conclusion?
- Share revised draft with peers.
- Invite correction of grammar, spelling, punctuation, usage.
- Incorporate corrections in final draft.

Final Draft

- Share the final product with peers.
- Invite evaluation.
- Have someone you know well read your essay. As they are reading, if they nod and smile in recognition, then you have a winner! You have successfully communicated who you are in a narrative. Congratulations!

That was a lot of work! The good thing is you can use all these steps when you write papers in college so keep these helpful hints with you. Put your essay aside for now. Let's take a look at letters of recommendation.

LETTERS OF RECOMMENDATION

Now it is time to have other people write about how well you would fit into the program you are applying to. At the end of Chapter 3, you had an opportunity to write your own letter of recommendation. That is the best way to understand the content that you need to go into a letter. If you have not done the exercise on page 78 yet, this is a good time to try it out. From writing your essay, you also know better what the school is looking for from reviewing their mission statement, philosophy, and essay focus. With this knowledge, you are in a good position to let your letter writers know what to emphasize in their recommendations. The more guidance you give to the people you ask for recommendations, the more likely you are to get what the school is looking for. When students ask me to write a letter of recommendation, I always ask the student to send me a description of the program that they are interested in so that I can write a letter that meets the needs of the students and addresses how the student will shine in their program.

The application may state who they want to have write letters of recommendation: a teacher, an employer, or someone in health care. Read the directions carefully. If the school does not indicate who they want to hear from, you can assume it is a teacher, a boss, or a mentor. Even though teachers have written many letters for students, it is still important to let the teacher you choose know the specific interests of the program. If you have been out of school for a while and you are asking a teacher from your sophomore year, it would be good to make an appointment with your former teacher to let them know what you have been up to since you were in their class. For those who have graduated and are coming back to school, you may consider letters from the professors who are teaching the prerequisite courses. That would mean that you are going to have to take the initiative to have the professors get to know you. It is possible. I just got an e-mail from a prerequisite course professor in microbiology telling me how outstanding the nursing applicant was.

Think of this request for letters from a writer's perspective. Although every year I work to know the hundreds of students I teach, it becomes difficult to write anything but a generic letter if I have not seen the student in a year, unless I have some prompts from the student. One way to update your recommender is to include your résumé with the request for a letter. See Chapter 6 for everything you need to write an outstanding résumé.

Most programs are going to want to know about your community participation, your leadership abilities, your intellectual curiosity, and your ability to relate to people because that is the kind of nurse our health care system needs: a smart leader who works well on a team and can relate to a variety of people. So you are going to want to ask the person who can write about you in those terms, right? Some schools give specific information in their directions as to what they need the recommender to speak to such as your strengths and weaknesses, how you measure up compared to other students and your future potential as a nurse. You may want to discuss these points and share some specific examples with your recommender so that they know your view. This is all to say that you have more control over this process than you may think. It is not like when you were younger and you handed a request to a family friend to write about your upstanding character. So you want to be thoughtful about letters of recommendation. The Admissions Committee's job is to compare your letters with those of other students so you want your letters to work in your favor.

Some schools have a numeric scale for letter writers to rate the applicant on oral communication, writing ability, leadership maturity, and social skills. So you will want to ask people who know you well enough to rate you on these scales. Make sure they know about the side of you that has these skills because you do not want them to put N/A, "not applicable." N/A does not tell the Admissions Committee what they want to know. Schools may ask the recommender to state how you will succeed in the program and to assess your future as a nurse. So, here is how you start:

1. Make a list of potential recommenders.
2. Narrow your list to the top three.
3. Let the top three choices know as soon as possible.
4. Give them 3 to 4 weeks to respond but also follow up so that your request does not get lost in their "to-do" file.
5. Send the recommendation form in a large envelope so that it does not have to be folded.
6. Send the instructions for writing the letter.
7. Let the recommender know they can contact you any time if they need more information.

8. Enclose your résumé (see Chapter 6 for résumé writing).

9. Send a stamped envelope for the letter to be sent directly to the school.

10. Know when the letter is due so that you can call or e-mail a reminder. I am asked to write many letters. It is helpful to have reminders.

11. A couple of days before the letter is due, write a thank you note to the recommender. That will be one more reminder and genuine words of appreciation to your recommender for taking the time to construct a letter that is going to get you to your preferred future!

The application checklist (Figure 4-2) can help you keep track of critical application information.

Affordability

Most schools list their costs on their Web sites. Make a list and compare tuition, fees, housing, program expenses, and length of program. Questions to address:

- Are there tuition reimbursement programs where you sign an agreement to work at a certain facility for a specific amount of time for free tuition?
- Can you expect to work during school? Some programs discourage employment, in others students work 2 to 3 jobs.
- Are there work-study programs?
- Is there an opportunity to be a teaching assistant for money or credit?
- Is there an opportunity to be a research assistant for money or credit?
- Should you look into being a Certified Nursing Assistant (CNA)? An Emergency Medical Technician (EMT)?
- Can you work in the hospital as a Student Nursing Assistant (SNAP) during the program?
- What financial aid is available?

Financial assistance comes in many forms, from federal loans to local town scholarships designated specifically for students in nursing programs.

Application Checklist

School of Nursing

Application deadline

Financial Aid deadline

Components of application	Sent	Received
Transcripts		
Essay		
Letters of recommendation		
1.		
2.		
3.		
Resume		

Financial Aid Packet

Figure 4-2. Application checklist.

Loans, grants, work-pay-back, scholarships, and work-study funding are financial assistance possibilities. Many financial support programs are need-based with eligibility determined by the Federal Need Analysis Methodology. Here I will give a broad overview of options. There are many books that address financial aid that give the specific details of each program. Before you start searching, contact the school's financial aid office for information and assistance with financial aid.

Financial aid can provide support for tuition, housing, books, and sometimes child care. In nursing school, students are also responsible for providing uniforms, laboratory fees, malpractice insurance, necessary equipment, and transportation to off-campus laboratory locations. The final state licensing exam costs approximately $350, plus the cost of the exam review course. These required expenses can add up. Consider them carefully.

These are the basics you will need to begin to apply for financial aid:

a. The school financial aid application

b. The Free Application for Federal Student Aid (FAFSA)

c. Your recent federal income tax returns

d. If applicable, registration card and other immigration documents

Federal and State Assistance

The FAFSA application is online at http://www.fafsa.ed.gov. There is a worksheet available that you can fill out before working electronically so that you will be ready with all the information you need to submit the application. You will need a Personal Identification Number (PIN) to apply electronically and submit the FAFSA forms (http://www.pin.ed.gov). After submitting the FAFSA forms, you will receive a Student Aid report (SAR) from the U.S. Department of Education. Review your information carefully and list the school you are applying to receive your information. The due date for the FAFSA forms is generally March 1, but check the web site and also the date for state financial aid. Table 4-1 summarizes federal aid and state scholarships.

Many schools have internal scholarships, some based on merit and others based on need. The **Nursing Reinvestment Act** provides scholarships to qualified undergraduate students (http://bhpr.hrsa.gov/nursing/scholarships.htm). The **Foundation of the National Student Nurses Association** awards undergraduate scholarships.

Local Assistance

Some towns, local hospitals, and churches offer scholarships to nursing students. To locate these specific scholarships may require a little research on your part but you may be surprised with what you come up with. At

Table 4-1. Federal Aid and State Scholarships

Federal Pell Grant	The Pell grant is for undergraduate students who have extreme financial need and who meet the strict eligibility requirements.
Federal Supplemental Educational Opportunity Grant (SEOG)	The SEOG is for undergraduate students with financial need who are enrolled full time.
Federal Perkins Loan	Priority for this 5% interest rate loan program is given to students with financial need. Repayment begins 9 months after the students are no longer enrolled at least half time. There are provisions for borrowers who work in qualifying health care facilities.
Federal Nursing Student Loan	Similar to the Federal Perkins Loan: 5% interest, no payback for student, until attending school less than half time based on financial need.
Federal Direct Loan	Schools participate in various federal loan programs. Check with the school office.
Federal Parent Loan for Undergraduate Students (PLUS)	This program is for parents of dependent undergraduate students. There is a variable interest rate adjusted every July 1.
Federal Work Study Program (FWS)	On-campus, part-time employment for students who demonstrate financial need.
State Scholarships	Each state offers grants and scholarships. Some are targeted specifically for nursing students. Visit your state website.

one time, many community hospitals had their own nursing school where there were nursing scholarships. Although the school has closed, nursing student scholarship money may still be available.

Some schools have specific grants to support nursing education and there may be individual faculty with research grants that hire undergraduate research assistants. Hospitals within your school's community may offer work-to-pay-back loan programs, where the hospital will pay student loans back if the student agrees to work at the facility for 2 to 3 years following graduation.

For complete assistance with financial aid, contact the schools' Financial Aid office.

THE CAMPUS VISIT

A student who visited our school recently observed that the key to finding the right fit between you and the school is to research the school thoroughly and then take a road trip to the school. The feeling you get from visiting a school means a lot to your decision. The chemistry between you and the faculty, the student tour guide, or the friendliness of people in the hallway will give you an idea of what the school is like. If you visit a couple of schools, you will really see and feel the difference. Consider visiting the school before you apply. That way you will not waste your money on application fees to schools you have no interest in. Some schools provide the opportunity to interview. I know what you are thinking; an interview does not exactly sound like a fun opportunity. But consider meeting with Admission Committee members as another way to let them know who you are and to demonstrate your passion for nursing. An interview is like an essay; you get to tell your story. In fact, some interviews are based on the essay. The interviewer will have you go more into depth on topics in your essay. So let's talk about turning the interview into an opportunity.

When first thinking about an interview, it seems like the whole scene is in the control of the interviewers. After all, they ask the questions, right? Actually, there is a lot you can do to prepare for an interview. If you think about it, you can guess what questions you may be asked and prepare your response ahead of time. That's what we will work on in the next section.

THE INTERVIEW

The first step to taking control of your own interview is to try to find out how many people will interview you so you can be prepared for a one-on-one interview or a group interview. Next, find out who the interviewers will be: will there be members of the Admissions Committee? Students? Faculty? If you know the players you can think of questions you might like to ask each individual. We'll practice this, too. When you call the school to arrange an interview appointment, ask if there is a format for the interview and areas that the interviewers will be most interested in. Some places will send you the interview questions. If there is no format then you have to anticipate the questions. The interviewers will probably ask you questions similar to the essay:

- Why do you want to be a nurse?
- Are you interested in a particular area of nursing?
- Tell us about your school career thus far.
- Tell us about a stressful situation and how you handled it.
- Tell us about (whatever their mission is) diversity, community, critical thinking, caring and leadership.
- Do you anticipate going to graduate school? (I am not kidding: this will be a question if you are applying to a university. See Chapter 7 to get a preview of graduate school so you have a clue as to what they are asking you).

Reflection 3: Prepare Your Answers

So let's try it. In response to these questions, you will need an example to go with each answer. Write a few points down now and consider writing the whole answer out before you go on the interview. Writing will help you think your answers through. It is good to be prepared because on the day of the interview you will be nervous.

1. Why do you want to be a nurse?

2. Tell us about your school career thus far.

3. Tell us about a stressful situation and how you handled it.

4. Tell us about (whatever their mission is) diversity, community, critical thinking, caring, leadership, and so on.

5. Tell us about your strengths as a student and tell us about what you think you can improve.

6. Who has been most influential in your learning?

When you think these answers through, you will be much less anxious about the interview. During the interview, there will be time for you to ask questions so make sure you have a few questions prepared. Remember that you are being compared to other applicants, so you want to have good questions to ask. For example: what would you like to know about the school, about the classes, about being in the clinical area? You can actually take every area the school is interested in and ask how you will be prepared to:

- Enter the diverse world of health care.
- Be a leader in nursing.
- Create a therapeutic relationship (that is what we call the professional connection with patients as oppose to a friendly relationship).
- Collaborate with health care team members.
- Use critical thinking in nursing.

You should practice for the interview like you are going to give a presentation. In preparation for a presentation it is helpful to:

- Identify your worst fear.
- Envision what success looks like.
- Identify three main points.
- Consider what will you say when you can't answer a question.
- Practice, practice, practice.

Reflection 4: Dress rehearsal

- Identify your worst fear about your interview.
- Envision what the interview will look like when you are doing well. What it will be like in the interview room? I mean really envision by picturing

yourself answering questions with confidence, picture the interviewers smiling and nodding. Take a few minutes to envision an interview where you nailed it!

- Identify three main points that you want to communicate in the interview. Chances are, if you know what you want to talk about you will find an opportunity to do so. Trust me.

- Consider what will you say when you can't answer one of the interviewer's question. That actually maybe a fear, but of course you will be able to answer all of the questions because the interview is about getting to know you. This is NOT a test. You just need to practice so that you are prepared to talk about you with more than one-word or one-sentence answers.

  — What stories will you tell to give examples of leadership, caring, and so on?

  — What will you say when they ask about your strengths and weaknesses? List your strengths and weaknesses.

  — How can you expand on the content of your essay?

- Practice, practice, practice. Just like giving a speech, you can practice for the interview. When you practice you will be so much more comfortable when the time comes.

FINALLY, WHAT TO WEAR TO THE INTERVIEW

You can wear your usual stuff when you are touring the campus but the interview will be different. Here you need to look like a business professional. This means you may have to shop for an interview outfit. The clothes you wear on an interview are not something that is in many high school closets. In the interview, how you look counts. That means NO super high heels, low camis, short skirts, sagging pants, tummy exposed. No sneakers, no jeans. Yes, for the men, a dress shirt and tie. You need to try on what you plan to wear, too, so that you will feel somewhat comfortable on the day of the interview. The night before the interview, just like your first day of school, lay all of your clothes out. This will also decrease last-minute anxiety that creeps in when you cannot find matching socks or a belt to wear. Take out piercings and hide tattoos. Think conservative, think business professional.

LAST, BUT NOT LEAST, WHAT IF?

What if you do not get in to nursing school? What next? This is worth thinking about so you have a Plan B. You always need a Plan B. Let's think about 10 hard questions:

1. Do you have backup schools?
2. Do you need to improve the grades you received in the prerequisite courses?
3. Will you apply to community colleges?
4. Will you look at private schools?
5. Will you go for a liberal arts baccalaureate degree and return as a second Bachelor's nursing student?
6. Can you take a year off? Will you work for a year between high school and college?
7. Can you work in health care?
8. Will you consider being a nursing assistant to get some valuable experience?
9. Was nursing the right choice for you?
10. What is another major that interests you?

Believe it or not, if you consider all of these questions, you will go into your application, essay, and the interview with more confidence because now you have a backup plan. Rejection will not feel good, but it will not be the end of the world. Not being accepted means that there are other things for you to do rather than nursing, or that nursing is a goal and you have to be better prepared to achieve that goal. If "what if" occurs, give yourself some time to regroup and then follow your dream no matter what?

CONCLUSION

The application essay and interview take preparation to do them well. You want to be prepared, organized, and confident. Preparation, organization, and confidence are attributes of successful students and excellent nurses.

The Admission Committee knows this. So your job is to demonstrate to the committee how well you will fit into nursing.

As you know from reading the chapter, none of this can be done on the fly. You need to map out a time frame and stick to it. You need to leave time for reflection, drafting essays and applications, and researching schools. Following a thoughtful process will set you apart from the other applicants and give you the competitive edge. In these days of wait lists to get into nursing schools, a competitive edge is exactly what you need!

Every student I have spoken with has said you can never be too prepared for nursing school. Going to a nursing class or walking into your first patient's room is always a shock. Chapter 5 brings you real-life experience from students on being successful in nursing school. Read on.

END-OF-CHAPTER EXERCISE

1. If you have not already done so, talk with students who are enrolled in the program you want to attend.

2. If you have already talked with students, then talk with a freshman, a sophomore, a junior, and a senior to get their different perspectives.

3. Talk with graduates of the program.

4. Talk with other practicing nurses and find out their recommendations.

References

Cameron, J. (1992). *The artist's way.* New York: G.P. Putnam's Sons.

Elbow, P. (1973). *Writing without teachers.* New York: Oxford University Press.

Elbow, P. (1981). *Writing with power.* New York: Oxford University Press.

Elbow, P. (2000). *Everyone can write.* New York: Oxford University Press.

CHAPTER 5

You're In!

How to Be Successful Once You Get There?

Congratulations! This is fantastic. You are going to be a nurse! This is so exciting to think about. If you just heard about your acceptance, then you are definitely into the first stage of role transition from a layperson to a nursing student. You have now entered the honeymoon stage. For every role transition, whether it is entering school or beginning a new job or even retiring at the end of a career, there are four stages of adjustment you'll go through. In this chapter, you will find out what to expect in transitioning into nursing school, you will hear the behind-the-scenes story from students about what they wish someone told them before they got there, you'll learn what you can do now to prepare for school, how to be organized and manage time once you get there, and you'll get an inside look at the clinical experience. We'll finish with how to manage the stress that comes with every program, take a look at the benefits of mentoring, and what is it like to be an older student in a traditional program.

Start at the beginning: Transition to a nursing student

1. Honeymoon
2. Shock/rejection
3. Acceptance
4. Assimilation

When you find out that you have been accepted into the nursing program, you will fly right into the honeymoon stage. When people are in this stage they are infused with energy; they are so excited they are moving faster than the speed of light. Everything looks rosy, the future is ripe with possibilities. I always hope when I am teaching a first-year course that the students will still be in the honeymoon stage. They will be upbeat, happy, thrilled to take on the job of studying to be a nurse. But, students tell me, "No way, we are over the honeymoon by the end of school orientation." In the orientation, students have been informed of the workload and what the life of a nursing student looks like. They are surprised at all the work that is going to be expected of them. By the time they reach their first course, they have moved into the "shock" stage. Of course, when they were applying to the program, they had heard from friends, "Oh, you are going to be a nursing student, you won't have a life." But they had no idea it would be this much work!

So enjoy the honeymoon and use your extra energy to get ready for school. You can begin to prepare yourself on your own by brushing up on health care issues in the local and national news. For example, in today's paper there was an article on the mystery of asthma, prenatal screening, and end-of-life care, all predominantly nursing care issues. You can learn about Healthy People 2010 (http://www.healthypeople.gov), check out the Institute of Medicine's work on patient safety (http://www. iom.edu/), and learn more about nursing education (http://www.aacn. nche.edu). It would be helpful to find out what books you will need for the first semester. No sense waiting around if you have time now. As one student responded when I asked how she succeeded in nursing school, "You have to be independent when you are in nursing, you have to rely on yourself." So you might as well start practicing now.

The second stage, "shock/rejection," is when you are shocked that you are required to read four chapters in pharmacology and there is a quiz every week, you have three chapters in pathophysiology to prepare for a class that is 3 hours long, you have two modules in health assessment that you need to memorize in order to demonstrate that you know how to assess for respiratory problems when you get to the lab, plus a written case study is due in ethics. You will know you are in the shock stage when your energy level takes a quick turn south and you lose your sense of humor. Nothing is funny. At this point, many students hit the couch. Those who sleep when they are anxious, now will sleep more; those who have a touch of insomnia when they are fearful, now will sleep less. Same with food. Those who get anxious and eat will start eating in this stage, those who get anxious and don't eat, that behavior will kick in. What you need to remember is that you are not alone. The Admissions Committee decided that you could succeed in school and that you will make a good nurse. So, you are in the right place even though things might seem a bit overwhelming. You are not dumb, you are not slow, you are not the only one who doesn't get it. A group of seniors recommended to new nursing students:

"Don't let the small things get to you."

"Just relax."

"Just do your work and you'll have nothing to worry about."

"Take a deep breath and calm down. Don't stress too much or you'll never get anything done."

"Find an older student to talk to."

In fact, the way to get through this stage is to talk to others in the program, find new friends, talk as a group. DO NOT isolate yourself and think you are the only one who is feeling stressed out and clueless. This is the phase during which successful students get together and complain to their new nursing friends. They talk about the work, long for the good old days, and find things wrong with the program they worked so hard to get into, "It is disorganized, faculty are insensitive, clinical starts too early, the nurses ignore students." This is normal. This is the rejection part of the shock stage. If you are an older student with a family, it would be wise to take time to hang out with your new younger peers. It is too stressful to go directly home and go through all of these feelings alone. The best thing to do is unite with classmates and remember it is only a stage. This, too, shall pass.

When the shock does decrease, you will be partway through school and beginning to find a place in the program you can live with. Not all faculty are as insensitive as you first thought; many of your teachers will be inspiring. Not all nurses ignore students, in fact most nursing students report that they love their nurse preceptors. You will figure out how to manage the workload or at least how to get by. This is the beginning of the third stage: "acceptance."

The acceptance stage can be recognized by the return of your sense of humor and the ability to manage your time, at least most days. You know that you are moving into accepting the nursing student role when you feel more comfortable participating in class and can voice some of the issues that you are concerned about rather than secretly harbor all those difficult feelings. In the clinical setting, you actually find nurses you want to emulate. You begin to have a hint that maybe you can do this. You have had experience with a patient that makes you feel like you can be a nurse. Lyndsay describes taking care of her patient in her third week of nursing school:

The first patient I met was an 84-year-old female, P.H. I expected to see this very disoriented, elderly woman when I arrived to do A.M. care. Turns out P.H. was doing much better. She was alert and very chatty. She was being discharged that afternoon to a rehab facility. The Technical Assistant helped her out of bed and prepared the bathroom for her to bathe. I watched but felt a little disappointed that I was not utilizing what I had learned. I laid out a pull sheet on the bedside chair, and eased P.H. into it. I sat on the bed next to her just to chat for a minute while my nurse brought another patient to surgery. Here I was sitting next to this tiny, old woman. Her hair was curled, and sticking up a bit from laying in bed. She did not look like someone who had fainted and fallen off a chair. She began to tell me her story and how foolish she had been. We all make mistakes, I assured her, it takes one accident to teach us. She was so concerned that her children had to deal with finding her a rehab facility, and the burden she had put on them. She spoke of her husband battling Parkinson's and she was the sole caretaker. This 84-year-old, petite lady was stronger than me, with a 63-year age difference. She was taking care of her husband, her home, and herself and worried about her children. P.H. reminded me what really matters in life. I was so worried about the physical aspect of nursing that I forgot I could be therapeutic by listening, and in the end she made me feel better, too.

Despite the rigors of the program, Lyndsay is committed to being a nurse, she has moved into the acceptance stage of socialization. The final stage, "assimilation," may happen toward the end of the program or after you graduate, when you begin to be more accomplished as a nurse. But before we get to the end, let's look at some research I did to find out what current nursing students wish they had been told before they started the program.

WHAT I WISH SOMEONE TOLD ME . . .

I asked ten focus groups of current students and recent graduates, "What do I wish someone had told me before I entered nursing school?" We talked about how to prepare for nursing school, what you need to know once you get there, and how you can manage your life in college. The first-semester students offered insightful and practical suggestions. We will learn about health care experience, organizational skills, and stress management. The students shared skills that you can begin learning right now. They recommended reading you can access and study skills you can practice. I also spoke with junior students in the midst of the program and senior students who had been through it all. We talked about how to manage clinical rotations, class requirements, and writing strategies. They suggested how to still have a social life, have a serious relationship, and keep your friends. I also had these students ask other students about managing difficult classes, giving class presentations, taking school exams, writing clinical journals, and dealing with faculty. Finally, we looked at managing stress and maintaining a healthy balance. Stay tuned for the inside story.

Starting with the first semester, nursing student's response to what I wish someone told me? Was immediately: "get some experience!"

Experience

Nursing is a hands-on profession and a hands-on education. In AD programs, you will be taking care of patients in your first semester. In BS programs, you will go from 2 years of liberal arts education to being in the hospital, on the unit, in the patient's room, taking care of a real person 2 weeks into junior year. Second Bachelor's students begin clinical the first 2 weeks of their first course. All students admitted that entry into the world of patient care is both exciting and challenging.

Here's what it is like as a new junior student, Megan writes:

On the first day of clinical, I was assigned to Mrs. S. I stood there outside her room, resmoothing my uniform, trying to decide how to go about introducing myself to this stranger. I had never done a bed bath or personal care for a patient before, and I suddenly felt sure that I would mess up this most basic of nursing tasks. I envisioned myself spilling water all over and the patient shivering with cold, or worse my inept hands somehow exacerbating her injuries or even breaking her frail body. It was as though all of my insecurities and deepest fears about being a nurse were suddenly focused on this moment, this patient. I had to physically take two steps backwards and reapproach the room. Just go in. "Don't think about it anymore," I told myself. I stepped into the room and approached Mrs. S's bedside.

Mrs. S was lying back, with her eyes barely open. Though it was morning, her face wore a pained wince and she looked utterly exhausted with beads of sweat matting a few straight gray hairs down onto her forehead. Her sheets and blanket lie in disarray, wadded up around her, and a sour smell laced the air. Obviously, Mrs. S was neither comfortable nor rested. Again, my fears welled up. Would this woman trust me to help her? What if she refused to let me near her? Would she know I had never done this before? "Good morning," I announced, unsure of the volume of my voice in the darkened room, "I'd like to help you get washed and dressed for breakfast." To my surprise, Mrs. S responded not irritably or warily, but cheerfully. "Oh, good morning! Thank you, I'd like that." Suddenly, the nagging thoughts of imagined failure retreated as I focused on the very real needs of this ill woman.

Megan was a junior in college when she started her first clinical. So even after 2 years of classes, starting the nursing program with nursing clinicals was still brand new. Although many students are like Megan and do fine with their clinical care, respondents to the "what I wish" question still said, "If you can get some experience prior to entering nursing school you will feel more confident with patient care and more comfortable when you start nursing classes and clinical." Student after student echoed Jenna's wish:

I wish I had known that working in a hospital prior to coming to school would have been beneficial. I actually did volunteer and did a high school internship at a hospital maternity ward but I wish I became a Certified Nursing Assistant (CNA) so I had clinical patient experience.

Jeff comments:

If I could go back, I'd have done more volunteering so I could have a sense of how things run.

Courtney recognizes:

It would have been good to know any sort of hospital experience would have been helpful. I had my first clinical last week and students in the group that were CNAs (certified nursing assistants) definitely had a step up from those of us who had never set foot in a hospital before. I looked around the unit and had no idea what anything was. However, those that had been in the hospital setting looked a lot more at ease because they came in with a certain skill set while the rest of us started out with a blank slate.

Courtney wisely adds

I'm sure it will all even out but it's always helpful to take the opportunity to do something that'll make you feel more comfortable.

Courtney is right, those familiar with a hospital setting will be less stressed and more comfortable. Volunteering is good, being a nurse's aid is better. In fact, some top schools have recognized that prior health care experience is so important for nursing students that in order to apply, the school requires volunteer or paid work. The University of Washington, one of the premier nursing schools in the country, states in the admission requirements:

It is expected that applicants have a minimum of 100 hours of volunteer or paid health care experience in one setting for a minimum of 3 months. Prospective students should note that a majority of competitive applicants have several hundred hours of health care experience for nine months or more.

In addition, an admission requirement is:

A letter of recommendation from a recent supervisor, preferably a registered nurse, who has supervised you in a paid or volunteer position in a health care setting. http://www.son.washington.edu

So, what are you waiting for? I know, you have had the same summer job throughout high school, you make good money, and you are familiar with the job requirements. Been there. I was a lifeguard in high school and volunteered in a hospital. I was comfortable with both jobs and I was really shy. Hours were good, got a tan . . . but that was not enough! It took me until between junior and senior year to bite the bullet. I recognized the same thing Courtney did. In our first clinical experiences in junior year, those students who had worked in a hospital knew the routines, were familiar with the equipment, and were more comfortable around patients, were better prepared. The students with experience could focus on the new skills and they could connect what they read in their textbooks to their experience; whereas I was reading in a vacuum. I did not have the real experience to see how our reading was relevant to actual patient care. Whether applying to school or in prenursing or already in the nursing program, experience in health care will prepare you for your future. One student who was going into her senior year came into my office, asking, "Shall I keep my job as a nanny this summer or work in a hospital? I make so much money as a nanny." I just sat quietly for a few minutes and she said, "I should work in a hospital, right?" By the end of our meeting, she actually figured out how to do some nannying and mostly hospital work.

Experience will build confidence. By feeling more acclimated to a health care situation you will be able to concentrate on your current learning rather than be preoccupied with the unfamiliar environment. With experience, all the equipment in a hospital and nursing homes won't be so foreign. You will know how to take a blood pressure, you have heard patients in pain, you have talked to patients who feel all alone. As a nursing assistant you would have probably sat in on a shift report, which means you have been in the staff room, behind the nurses station, where visitors cannot go. With experience you have seen the machines around a patient's bed. You have probably watched a nurse conducting a patient assessment, witnessed a nurse giving a patient treatment, or seen the nurse passing medications. When you have a job as a nurse's aid and the nurses know you are going into nursing school, they will often take you under their wing and explain more about patient care. This type of mentoring is invaluable.

It takes time and money to be a Certified Nursing Assistant (CNA), but I have heard over and over again that it is time and money well spent. Nursing assistants get to spend time with patients. I won't paint a rosy picture. The CNA job is not easy. CNAs get to interact with patients, often more than the nurse does. They bathe and feed patients, help patients walk, and assist in prescribed exercise. CNAs form important therapeutic relationships with patients. All of these skills, bathing, walking, and relating, you will learn as a beginning nursing student. You will be so much less stressed, though, if you have already taken care of patients, carried out nursing tasks, and functioned as a member of a health care team. In this narrative, Leah, a CNA at the time, describes one of the patient relationships she developed:

Anna was a small woman—about 5'4" or so. She had dark hair, graying and thinned by age. Deep circles surrounded dark eyes, carved out above high cheek bones. Her shoulders were stooped and she could only take a few steps with assistance. When I first met her she could transfer out of bed by herself, though she seldom left her room. Though there was no official diagnosis, the staff had labeled Anna as having obsessive compulsive disorder because she had a very specific routine for personal care. She spent a lot of time washing and combing her hair so that it lay perfectly flat against a pale, shiny scalp. She liked to eat by herself in her room; her roommate went to the dining room.

As the months passed, Anna became more and more debilitated. After a bad fall while transferring from the toilet, she could no longer physically care for herself. I, as her nursing aide, became deeply involved in her care—helping her to wash and dress, applying toothpaste to the brush and helping her into bed. Anna was very specific about the way washing should be done. Clothing should never touch the floor. She needed several Kleenex laid underneath her nightgown before she went to sleep. Her hair must be combed flat even when she was about to climb into bed. Instructions were conveyed in choppy Spanish, a language I had a limited grasp of.

After she was in bed and comfortable, I would sit on the safety mat on the floor beside her bed and we would talk. She told me about immigrating to the United States from Columbia. Though she never went into detail when I asked, she grimaced when talking about Columbia. "Muy duro," Very hard, *was her commentary on her childhood. She had met her husband in the United States. He was shorter than her, she said with a grin. I laughed and replied that my own partner was shorter than me, too. Anna's husband had passed away years before.*

Anna spoke about her daughter, a woman deeply troubled by mental illness. The daughter rarely came to visit, though her husband and son (Anna's nieto *or* chiquito) *came to visit once in a while. Anna held the little boy on her lap and smiled widely for the entire time they stayed. My conversation with Anna always ended with a hug and kiss. "Te quiero, Anna,"* I love you, *I would say.*

One afternoon I came into work and during report I was told that Anna had had a stroke. The entire left side of her body was paralyzed. Anna was, of course, devastated. Thinking that I was helping her to cope with the new disability, I replied that she would get strong again. Each time I came into work she would show me the exercises she had been doing. After weeks of practice, she could lift her left leg about an inch from the mattress. She could tense the thigh muscle. Also, Anna was intent on keeping her right arm strong. She did exercises in bed at night.

Then, Anna broke her right wrist and it was discovered that Anna had a rare bone disorder. She was in constant pain. She could no longer transfer to the toilet without an electronic hoyer lift. She stopped being able to wait to go to the toilet and became incontinent of urine. Later, she became incontinent of stool.

Somewhere along the line Anna gave up. She finally asked me, will it ever get better? She gestured to the left side of her body. I shook my head, no. She was beyond rehabilitation, I thought to myself. She would spend the rest of her life confined to a broad chair. After that, Anna's mental health began to deteriorate. My conversations with Anna became guessing games. Her speech was incomprehensible at times, muddled with words of her own creation. Sometimes she appeared to be having hallucinations and would refer to things that I could not see, gesturing and picking at the air. I sat with her after she was in bed or on my break, holding her hand and listening to a barrage of language I could no longer understand. I felt as though a part of her had died. Where had my friend gone? Anna no longer laughed or smiled—a constant grimace on her face.

Anna now lives on the dementia unit in the nursing home that I work. We don't talk the way we used to. I have a hard time sitting with her now; find myself completely drained just by being near her. I go downstairs to say hello and hold her hand. She recognizes me to this day, but cannot speak anymore. I wonder sometimes if she thinks that I've abandoned her, that I stopped loving her and wanting to take care of her.

As you can hear, Leah played a very important role in Anna's care. There is no question that in this situation the care was good the patient and good for Leah's future as a nursing student.

Another advantage of being a CNA is you will know what it is like to be delegated tasks. You will see what type of delegation skills work. When you are a nurse you will need to delegate to the CNA and it is helpful to have been on the other side. Experiencing what works with delegation and what does not work is very good to know as a nurse. Garrett, who had been a nurse's aid, wrote:

I feel my experience as an aid will give me the logic to delegate with aides without getting them too angry or expecting too much from them.

With experience not only have you already been responsible for nursing tasks but you have also worked with different types of patients. You have seen different kinds of nurses, those nurses who serve as role models, and those nurses who are not what you aspire to be like. You have observed the nurse-patient relationship, nurse-nurse relationships, and nurse-physician relationships. With experience, you will have prepared yourself for the incapacitating illness that patients present with. Witnessing human frailty can be difficult. Debra, a student new to the health care environment, wrote:

Though I have heard stories and watched movies about patients with altered mental status, chronic diseases and just poor quality of life, it is not the same as being there. When I worked on a floor for our first clinical and saw patients that were stuck in wheel chairs, moaning in pain and not able to get out of bed by themselves, my heart broke. I felt like I couldn't swallow and was becoming teary eyed. All of this from just seeing a patient. I wish I could have had more time to prepare myself to deal with these feelings.

With previous health care experience, you will still have some of the feelings Debra is describing, but you will have had time to integrate those feelings so when you step onto a unit you will be a bit more prepared.

Before rushing out to your local hospital unit, why not read about what to expect so you can formulate some ideas about what you want to learn. If you have some knowledge about what nurses are reading and writing about, when you call about jobs, you will have idea about where you might like to work.

Now, this part is fun. This is the time to get in and find out more about what nurses think about, what they research, and what they write about. This information will make you so proud of the field you are going into.

The books listed at the end of Chapter 1 are a good place to start to learn about nursing. In addition, you can read clinical cases and research reports that nurses publish in professional nursing journals. Leah, a new nursing student, observes:

I wish I had read more nursing journals and nursing books to hear about other nurse's experiences so I had something to relate to. It would make it easier for me so if I am ever in the same situation I can read back to what they wrote and get an idea how to handle it.

You *can* go to your local college community college or hospital library and read professional nursing journals. Yes, you are allowed to do this. Some of my favorite people are librarians in small community hospitals because they are so helpful. Even if you are in high school you can go into the hospital library and talk to the librarian. Chances are the librarian would be delighted to show you the nursing journal section. I guarantee you will be amazed at how many different journals there are and I am sure you will find one you would like to read. So choose a few journals, grab a comfortable chair, and dive in. You can also get a taste of the nursing world by reading articles from journals on line. Check out http://www.ajn.online to see what's up.

The library will also have nursing textbooks. The college bookstore will have the textbooks students are currently using. Might as well take a look, soon you will be living and breathing the content in your nursing books. You can read what nursing students need to know right now. You can trek into the university where the reference librarian is waiting to assist you. Through your research into the world of nursing you will become somewhat familiar with what is going on in health care. You will learn about all the different topics nurses research and report their findings on. You will find topics from postpartum depression to women and cardiac disease to developing a day program for the chronically mentally ill. You will probably be drawn to certain topics that may give you an idea which area of nursing you may be interested in.

From your research, you will have more knowledge of the world of nursing care. Considering the majority of students come in thinking of *Scrubs* and *Grey's Anatomy*, it is to your benefit to find out what is really going on in nursing. After you are more familiar with what nurses are studying, then you should pick up the phone and call your local hospital, nursing home, or medical center and find out how to get some experience. Every health care facility needs more staff to care for patients. They will be happy to hear from you. In fact, when you do begin a job in a hospital you may hear about scholarships to school or loan programs that are designed to support students in school for the promise of working in that facility for a year or two after graduation. There are many benefits from gaining health care experience.

Once you have a job, the experience will help you learn how to organize your time to meet the job responsibilities. Many students wrote about the importance of developing organizational skills and time management techniques before they got to their clinical year so they are ready to combine class work and clinical responsibilities. You can start developing organizational skills right now.

Organization

Think about how you organize your time. How do you fit in school, studying, sports, and a social life? Student after student report that learning how to manage their time to be better organized would have really helped with the amount of work that is required in nursing. Michael admitted:

I did not realize how much time I had to put in each class. In high school I just breezed by, never really studying, always getting good grades. Now I have to work my behind just to pass some classes, never mind getting an A.

Students told me they need to create a schedule that is good enough to complete all their school work, readings, and studying *and* they wish they had started learning how to manage their time in freshman year.

The list of the ten basic organizational skills are going to seem obvious but even graduate students say they wish someone had handed them a list of "must haves" so that they could be more prepared. So here are your basic ten:

Ten "must have" organizing tools

1. Notebook for each class
2. Dividers and notebook paper
3. Three-hole punch
4. Stapler
5. Highlighters
6. Index cards, lots of index cards
7. Date book
8. Calendar
9. Computer
10. Printer

A computer and printer are nice to have, but they are also available in the library and probably in the nursing lab. Schools make every effort to have the equipment students need accessible and available. You just need to find out where and when the computers are available. So here is how nursing school works:

On the first day of each course, you will receive a course outline that has a course description, the course objectives, books required, readings recommended and the topic for each class with due dates for each assignment. Once you have the course outline, the next step is to:

1. Take that hole punch and put your outline into the notebook for that class.
2. Highlight the assignment due dates.
3. Mark the due dates in your date book and on your calendar.
4. Buy the required text books.

For each course, follow the same four steps until you have each course outline in its own notebook and each assignment due date on the calendar. Sometimes different classes require assignments due on the same day.

If you notice this in the beginning of the semester and bring the information to the faculty often due dates can be changed. It is more difficult to change due dates as the semester moves on, so it is better to organize up front. Some students find it useful to color-code each class so you can keep track of assignments by color. The key is to keep that calendar in front of you. Yup, I know that calendar looks overwhelming, but remember, you were admitted to the program because the faculty think you can make it and you can! Suzy writes:

Honestly, doing things like making lists and having binders, and just basically being organized helps me from freaking out.

There's a voice of experience. Once you know when the assignments are due you need to do some time management. You need to learn the art of back-planning or starting from the due date and working backwards.

Appendix A, at the end of the book, is a list of sample assignments required in an introductory nursing course.

Back-Plan

Back-planning is starting when the assignment is due, whether it is a paper or a quiz and working backward from the due date. Back-planning will give you the time and organization to study and retain information. As Kate reminds us:

As juniors we have to seriously understand what we learn because it's for real now. We can't forget the information once we take the test because people's lives are in our hands.

To learn and retain new information you will have to go beyond the infamous college all-nighters. To retain the information past the test or write a decent paper, the all-nighter does not really work. In addition, you will want to remember the information that you are getting in nursing classes so that you will know how to take care of patients. So you need to organize your time. Here is an example of back-planning:

Let's say you have a paper due October 10, five weeks after you start classes. Plenty of time. Or is it? For the paper you are going to have to find academic articles to pull information from to support the points in your paper. Finding academic articles means you are going to have to learn how to search the library database (you can learn the necessary skill of database searching now). Any references librarian can coach you in information literacy. Chances are your college library has instructions online on how to find current literature, but if you are like most of us you will want to take a trip to the library to meet with the reference librarian. That is their job, to coach students, so do not feel shy about this. Plus, it is much easier being guided by an expert on your first try.

Okay, so you need to access the literature. Whether you do it on your own or consult with the librarian, searching the literature will take time. So let's back up a day or two, at the minimum, from the due date to October 8. My librarian friend warns me that it takes 75% of the time to find the information you need and 25% to write the paper. I am not so sure a paper comes together that fast but I found his words to be comforting in that it takes time to locate the information you are searching for. Once you locate the literature you need you have to copy it, read it, highlight the important points, take notes and interpret what this article is saying. That will take a day or two or three. Back up to October 5. Once you have figured out what the literature is saying you have to begin to write your paper. To go through the five stages of writing your paper you will need a minimum of three days for:

1. Prewriting
2. Drafting
3. Editing
4. Second draft, revise
5. Final draft

Back up to October 2. Now you will need to type your paper, make revisions, cite the paper properly in American Psychological Association (APA) format. You probably used Modern Language Association (MLA) citation system in high school as a way to site information from articles so that you did not plagiarize. In nursing school, the APA format is preferred. So to type the paper, revise your writing, and cite the sources let's back up a day or two, at least to October 1. So now you know that if your paper is due October 10 that you will have to start the paper by October 1, that's if you do something on your paper every day, don't take a weekend off, and stay focused. Put that start date, October 1, on your calendar and watch your stress decrease. You will feel much less anxious once you have a plan and have scheduled the time to follow that plan. In addition, if you know your topic well in advance you will begin to see information for your paper as you go through your day. For example, *you decide to write a paper for the Ethics class on end-of-life care and lo and behold there is an article in the weekend newspaper on palliative care or as you are surfing the net you notice an item on health care proxy. Having information for your paper will contribute to your organization and lower your stress level. Promise.*

You can back-plan for a quiz, a test, or a care plan. Mark the date of the quiz on your calendar and judge when you are going to have to start studying. The night before is not the correct answer. Peter writes:

I think it would have been very helpful if someone had told me how difficult it was to manage your time. With my course load, clinicals every week, having a job, and participating in extra curricular activities I find myself in a daze, never knowing what is done and what isn't.

Shannon created an Excel back-plan and sent it to all of her peers to help them organize by back-plan. Figure 5-1 is an example of a back-plan prepared by a nursing student.

With organizational strategies we will know how to get the job done. There is no question that managing your life will be a juggling act, but it would be better to think of your schedule as a balancing act and develop skills to keep your life in balance.

Peter goes on to say:

If I had known it was going to be this bad then I would have never joined club softball or football, I would have not made my work schedule working over 15 hours/week.

Working and extracurricular activities, however, do not need to be ruled out. You just need to plan, organize, and prioritize. I have had several college athletes do well in nursing. There was a first-string ice hockey player who made every practice and traveled the entire East Coast to play games. There was a varsity volleyball player who traveled, a crew member who trained before 7 A.M. clinicals, and a varsity football player who never missed a practice or a class. I have had students with one, two, and three jobs. Julie and Alison were excellent students. I know these students because they also volunteered to be undergraduate teaching assistants in addition to working in the cafeteria and being a nanny. It is possible to be a successful nursing major and have an active college life. Elizabeth, in her freshman year, was worried that with her learning style she would not be able to focus on all

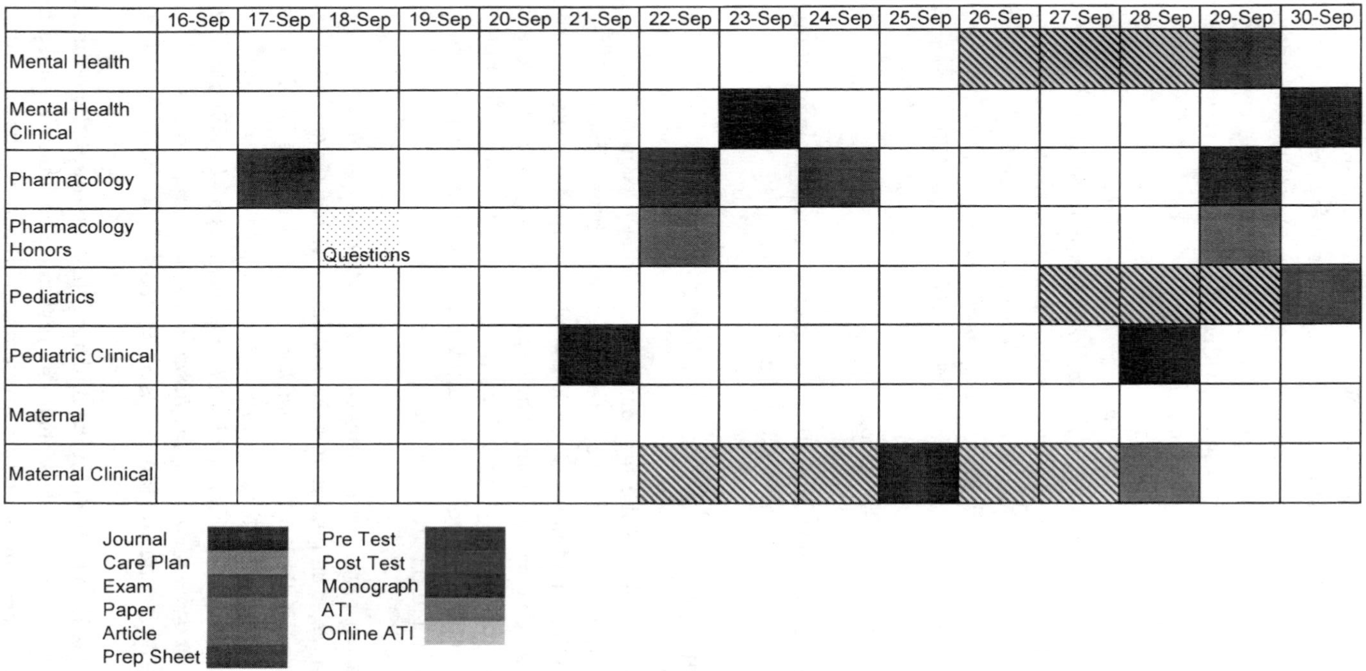

	16-Sep	17-Sep	18-Sep	19-Sep	20-Sep	21-Sep	22-Sep	23-Sep	24-Sep	25-Sep	26-Sep	27-Sep	28-Sep	29-Sep	30-Sep
Mental Health															
Mental Health Clinical															
Pharmacology															
Pharmacology Honors			Questions												
Pediatrics															
Pediatric Clinical															
Maternal															
Maternal Clinical															

Legend:

- Journal
- Care Plan
- Exam
- Paper
- Article
- Prep Sheet

- Pre Test
- Post Test
- Monograph
- ATI
- Online ATI

Figure 5-1. Page from a "back-plan" prepared by a nursing student.

there was to know about nursing. When I ran into her in her junior year, just as she was starting in clinical she was a manager at a local gym, an undergraduate teaching assistant, went on the cross-cultural trip to study with a midwife in the Dominican Republic, was doing great in her coursework, and was planning on graduate school. Evidently, the learning style she was concerned about fit well with nursing. It can be done. Katrina recognizes:

Nursing school is a big task to jump into. However if there is motivation and commitment, success will likely follow. When I was a senior in high school everyone told me how hard nursing school would be. Even now people say, "Oh you are in nursing school, you don't have a life outside of that." This is not true. Yes, this is a difficult, time consuming major, but if one budgets their time well, stays on top of their school work, they can still hang out on weekdays with friends and go out on weekends. I guess time budgeting and not stressing out are key points to know.

Recommendations from the front line: Keeping on top of school work, budgeting time, and not stressing out.

Keep on Top of School Work

In nursing, you know the first day of class what is required for the entire semester. Your course outline is your contract with the faculty. That is the good news. The bad news is you know what is due for the whole semester and that can be overwhelming. The key is to develop a calendar and budget your time. Just take the work bird by bird. Author Anne Lamott (1995) wrote about her younger brother attempting to complete an overwhelming project the night before it was due:

Thirty years ago my older brother, who was ten years old at the time, was trying to get a report on birds written he had had three months to write. [It] was due the next day. We were out at our family cabin in Bolinas, and he was at the kitchen table close to tears, surrounded by binder paper and pencils and unopened books on birds, immobilized by the hugeness of the task ahead. Then my father sat down beside him, put his arm around my brother's shoulder, and said, "Bird by bird buddy. Just take it bird by bird."

Students I have taught in the undergraduate program, the returning RN program, and the second Bachelor's program have found the bird-by-bird mantra very helpful. Doctoral students writing their dissertation repeat this story to incoming students. So let's take your school work one assignment at a time, bird by bird.

Once your notebook is organized and your calendar is filled in with due dates and you have identified the date you need to start each assignment, then you just need the commitment and motivation to stick to the plan. To keep your motivation up, just keep in mind that everything you are learning you will use as a nurse. As Kate acknowledged, "You will need to remember the information beyond the test so you can provide safe and competent patient care."

Fortunately, you will have the opportunity to put the classroom knowledge to work and practice your new nursing skills in the skills lab. Every nursing school has a skills lab with equipment and mannequins that you can practice your new skills on. With new technology, our equipment is becoming more realistic every day. Many schools have "Sim Man," which is a mannequin that has different sounds that mimic human features, such as a heart rate, lung sounds, bowel sounds, and the ability to talk to the nurse. The skills lab provides an excellent practice environment for students. Putting your book knowledge to work on Sim Man or practicing taking blood pressure on each other will help you recall the nursing skills, communication techniques, and patient interventions you read about in your text so you will be prepared to work with real patients. Making fun of their time in the lab, a group of students suggested the following title for a paper:

Nursing school is the only major where you have to take your clothes off for the midterm but you are not guaranteed an "A."

Very funny. Don't worry, though. You do practice some skills on each other in the lab, but you don't take your clothes off. Our midterm is conducting a health assessment on volunteer patients. Good practice for the real thing.

Budgeting Time

Every student will tell you that time management is the key. Budgeting your precious time is an essential skill to learn early:

I think that working and going to school was the hardest thing for me. It's just one more thing added to your long list of things to do. I remember working one night before my big physical assessment final last year. I only made like $20 that *night and lost so much time. When you have things like that in your schedule, you have to work that much harder to be organized. You have to manage time.*

So you really learn about time management.

Things like keeping a planner and just basically keeping up and staying on top of your work.

Students talked about feeling like they were in college but they were really working already because of their requirements and their schedule:

We have a Friday-Saturday clinical. We are getting into our car at 4 A.M. when people are stumbling into their dorms.

Thursday, thirsty Thursday, is the biggest night to go out here. We are finally 21 and we miss everything! We miss karaoke, we miss jeopardy. You cannot get trashed and think you can study pharm the next day. You definitely cannot go to clinical hung over. This major does affect you, majorly!

If you budget your time you will have time for friends. Not as much time as everyone else here, but some time.

No question, nursing is a serious major. Remember what I said in the first chapter though, the nursing students are the only students recruited for jobs in your first semester senior year! On top of the class work, there is the preparation that must be done for clinical. Clinical is when you go to the hospital or to a visiting nurses association to take care of patients. At first you shadow a nurse or nursing assistant and within a week or so you will be assigned your own patient. In some programs, to prepare for giving patient care, you are required to go on the night before and read your patients chart. One student told me:

You have to come as prepared as you can. It's not like you can prepare for clinicals like you can prepare for a class, but you have to do things like get a goodnight sleep and eat that morning. It makes a big difference.

Clinicals are what every student looks forward to. In clinical, you are in uniform, getting shift report from the nurses from the night before, and assigned to take care of a patient. You get to be like a real nurse. Patients, nurses, and physicians relate to you like you are the nurse. All nursing students cannot wait for clinical, then that day arrives and they are scared to death:

As I stood in the doorway, I thought that someone was going to have to come up to West Three in order for my feet to become unglued to the floor. As if the fear of being with a patient alone for the first time was not enough, the fact that she was MRSA precautious just added to it so I would have to get dressed in a long yellow gown gloves and a mask. I thought, "If I needed help quickly, it was going to be a good ten seconds before someone could don a gown, gloves, and mask," and I very well knew that ten seconds can feel like a lifetime in any emergency. After noticing I was the only navy blue and white scrubs left in the hall, I somehow managed to talk myself into thinking that this could be easy. As I was dressed in my gown, gloves and mask I approached the closed curtain and I felt like I was going to inspect a specimen rather than a patient in my get up.

Another student wrote:

The day started as I tried my hardest to contain the butterflies in my stomach—we were all going to get our own patient today. Besides the regular morning routine and care, we also got to try out new tasks: an injection or a dressing change. I was nervous and excited at the same time.

Different schools offer different types of clinical experience. Some programs assign eight students to one instructor and the students rely on the instructor for guidance. This is referred to as the duckling model, where students are trailing after the mother duck. One student writes:

Sometimes you can sit around for hours not doing anything waiting for your instructor. There will be time that you will feel lost and alone and not know what to do. If and when that happens, don't worry, you're not alone. I guarantee you that there are other people in your group that feel the same way.

Other teaching models place each student with a nurse preceptor called the clinical educator model or clinical faculty associates. This model can be difficult to execute with the staff nurses being so busy these days. But, it is great for students to be able to shadow a nurse. Garrett writes:

I had the opportunity to shadow an RN during my second clinical day. It gave me the opportunity to witness first hand the stresses and routine of a typical day as a nurse.

The nurse I was assigned to follow was a brand new nurse fresh off of orientation. It was literally his third day on his own, although he had been working on the floor as an aid for over two years. I was very impressed with his level of comfort and his organizational skills. He had already developed a routine that was very thorough.

We began the day with the preparation of the documents of the patients that he would be caring for throughout his day. He gathered supplies that he needed and received report from the nurses that cared for the patients on the previous shift. It was quite a bit more involved than I would have originally thought.

We next began to see the patients by starting at one end of the hallway, giving a quick introduction to each patient before going back to the beginning and performing 10-minute assessments. This took about 45 minutes to complete. Next, we started passing out medications. This consumed, literally, the next 3 hours without any time to do anything else. One of the patients had 18 medications that had to be taken by mouth. I can tell this is going to take the majority of my time.

Eighteen medications! And you have to know all of their treatment effects, their side effects, and their interactions. Now we are getting serious. In clinical, whether you are placed with faculty or a staff nurse, students insist:

You really can't be afraid to ask questions. It's important to find a nurse who you feel comfortable asking about things because they know all about the business and what you should and shouldn't do.

Another student chimes in:

It's important to find a nurse who can answer some of your questions. There is only one instructor and if you're taking up all of his/her time then your classmates are going to get angry and you don't want that because they have to be your support system.

Students recognize that they may have started out in cliques with each other freshman and sophomore year but by the time they were in clinicals every student must be your friend. One nursing student admitted:

In the prenursing classes everyone was in a clique, you found your people, drew the lines for the in-group and the out-group, then you get to clinical and you are placed in a clinical group with seven other students. Students you might not know, might not like but trust me, they will become your best friends.

I think you really rely on your classmates. It's not just about knowing and not knowing things. Sometimes you see things that bother you, scare you, make you worried. It's important to find someone there who is seeing the same things and going through the same exact things that you are going through.

I get through by relying on my peers. There is so much work to get through in nursing school. If you want to stay sane, you have to support each other and split up the work when it's possible.

Make friends with your peers. Make study groups so that you can get other people's perspectives on topics you are studying. Maybe they'll think of something totally different than you and bring ideas you never thought of to the table.

Peer support is essential to success. Remember the Shock stage of role transition? Well, here you are transitioning into clinicals and you need to go through it together. Some students are good at writing clinical journals, others are good at taking tests, some love to speak up in class, others come with clinical experience from being a CNA. You need each other to do well in school.

Seasoned students strongly recommend that you find a professor you can relate to. It helps to have someone who is "in the know" to go to with your questions and concerns. Sara, who was a very shy freshman who came from a small town to a large university, is now an outspoken senior:

Once you talk to one professor you are more likely to talk to others. And you have to speak up in clinical, you have to ask questions and state your needs so you can get the patient experience you need. Even though you are scared to death you have to step forward and volunteer to insert that catheter or change that dressing. That is the only way you will learn.

Come prepared to clinical with those questions:

You really can't be afraid to ask questions. It's important to find a nurse who you feel comfortable asking about things because they know all about the business and what you should and shouldn't do.

To succeed in clinical, you need to follow the principles of harmony and balance that Angeles Arrien (1993) suggests:

1. Show up and choose to be present—arrive at clinical on time, prepared to be actively present with patients and staff.
2. Pay attention to what has heart and meaning—this is the principle of the Healer, stop, look, and listen to the patient, work to understand what is meaningful to the patient.
3. Tell the truth without judgment—the patient defines their own health, but you can let the patient know your perception.
4. Be open to outcomes, not attached to outcomes—be aware of expected outcomes but be open to possibilities.

Michaela, a student nurse, intuitively knew to show up, be present, and let go of the outcomes:

Frank was a challenging character to figure out. He was the "sweet old man," the "pitied widower," and "depressed and suicidal" all in one. He was a frequent flyer on the mental health unit where the staff knew him to be expressive and creative. On the med/surg unit though, where we met, he was known as "attention seeking" and difficult to treat due to his chronic pain.

As a first semester nursing student I was at Frank's beck and call . . . and happily so. With every trip to Frank's room we talked about life "back when" and especially about his wife. Frank spoke affectionately about his care for Cynthia when she was in a long-term facility and how he used to iron her outfits each morning and bring them to her so that she could look "as beautiful as the day [they] were married." Clearly, ol' Frank was a catch. He shared detailed memories about the long boat trip to America from Scotland as a young boy, "One day, in the belly of the ship," Frank recalled, "my dad said, 'Frankie, get up on that table and sing and dance and make these people happy.' So I did. I was a little one but I just danced and danced, and I could sing too." Hearing these stories of care and being carefree, it was hard to imagine Frank attempting to take his life or suffering alone at home with chronic pain and no one to share his stories with. A quick look at his wrists and the freshly healed lacerations were a stark reminder.

Mid-way through my shift with Frank, the pain above his eye became intense. No need for the pain scale question here, it was clearly a 10. Nerve blocks and medications had been attempted in the past but couldn't touch this pain. Behind the curtain, holding Frank's hand as he groaned, I felt helpless. I also felt at ease. At ease enough to stay in touch with what used to comfort me as a kid. In an attempt to distract Frank from his pain I asked him to sing to me. "Do you remember any tunes from your days singing as a kid?" "Ohhh," he moaned. But he looked me in the eye with a glimmer of interest, of recollection. "I know some songs, Frank. Maybe you know this one." And I started to sing quietly. I sang, "Let me call you Sweetheart" and could tell he was listening. I tried another, "The Old Lamp Lighter." He was definitely listening. I tried another, and he was humming through his pain. We kept singing, together, little snippets of songs, humming when neither of us could remember the words. I smiled all the while and thanked my lucky stars that my weird parents had spent time singing old tunes in the car and around the kitchen table when I was young. I felt blessed with the sensitivity that could lead to this connection with Frank and for my parents who instilled it in me.

Frank's pain subsided but now he had found center stage. He kept on singing! Much to his roommate's chagrin he sang straight through to the following week when I returned. The nurses loved it though, and relayed to me that they found a different Frank after I left. Quietly, I was proud, and resolved to keep the "me" that I found with Frank even outside of the curtains on the frenzied floors and where ever else this new nursing adventure may take me.

Show up, be present, tell the truth, let go of outcomes. A mantra for clinical. For class and clinical you have to be ready to participate and in the midst of all this work you need to attend to yourself before you can attend to others.

Taking Care of Yourself: Stress Strategies

From all you have read so far, you get the picture: studying nursing is an important job, a high-pressured job, and a rewarding job. To be at your best, you need to manage the stress that comes with learning to be a nurse. You need to take care of yourself. Starting stress management routines in school will provide the self-care base you need to be successful in practice. Everyone has their own personal stress plan. Many stress plans have similar features. Think about it.

Reflection 1

1. What stresses you out now?

2. How do you manage stress now?

3. Do you see that strategy working in college?

Learning about managing stress as a nursing student has a double benefit: you will do better in school and with 80% of today's illness related to stress, you will be able to teach your patients about managing their stress. The stress strategies students suggested fell into five categories:

1. Take a break
2. Exercise
3. Vent
4. Diversion
5. Connect:
   a. Friends
   b. Family
   c. Faculty

Take a Break

As you know, there is a lot of work required to learn how to be a nurse, but you still need to take time for yourself. How can you care for others if you do not take care of yourself? One student writes:

It is important to still take time for yourself even if it is just relaxing watching TV or taking a bath.

Another student reiterates the importance of attention to self in the midst of the pressure:

You have to take time for yourself. There's no way around it, you just have to. Being a nursing student is part of you and if you don't take care of yourself there is no place for that nurse inside you to exist.

Wise words from experienced students. There are different ways to give yourself time away from work. One proven stress manager is to exercise.

Exercise

We know exercise helps to renew your energy, tone your muscles, and keep you in shape. We also know when you are tired you will feel better after you exercise rather than take a nap. Exercise gives you more energy, naps can tire you out. Students recommend:

Join a gym. Of course you can't afford it but ask for a membership for your birthday. In many gyms if you work the front desk for one shift you can work out for free. You have to workout, even it is just a walk.

I like to exercise. It relieves stress and makes me feel good about myself. I feel like if I just do something like watch TV, it's just a waste of my time and I get more stressed. I may as well be doing something that is good for me.

Exercise can help your body and your head. All those obsessive thoughts will quiet down to a dull roar so you can think again. A good exercise break can give you energy and make you feel more relaxed. Sometimes, you just need to talk or write about what you are experiencing.

Vent

It helps to vent. I usually vent to my peers. I usually feel better after that, but if I don't then I vent to my professors.

Talking with friends gets your worries out of your head and onto the table so others can listen to what you are thinking. First, you need to find a friend that can listen. Many find that other nursing students understand you best, others find someone outside of nursing is the most curious about your experience:

I think it helps to have friends that are nursing majors and friends who are not. Sometimes you need someone to understand exactly what you are going through and feels how you do. This is when it helps to have close friends in the program.

Talking to older students and practicing nurses can provide support:

I think it's important to talk to nurses at clinical and older students. They tell you exactly what you need to hear: it's hard, but you will make it through, just look at me. That's all you really want to hear, and it means more coming from someone who has survived.

Sometimes it's better to go to a professional counselor to listen to your concerns. College counselors have heard from many people your age and are experts in the problems college students face. In most college health clinics, you can go for a couple of sessions for free or for a minimal copayment. If you have not done this before, it is a real treat to have a counselor listen closely to you. Think of it this way: we religiously bring our car in for a tune-up, why not bring yourself in for a tune-up too?

Writing stresses down helps many practicing nurses so why not take a page from their book. My friend, Rozy, who is an orthopedic nurse, tells me she must come home and write about her day so she can sort things out, get in touch with what she is feeling and anticipate what to do next. Writing helps to leave things on the page so she can attend to her family. Julia Cameron, in *The Artists Way*, suggests writing three quick pages every morning so you can start the day with a clear head. Morning, night, after work, find out what works for you. Get yourself a journal, a pen that feels good, and give yourself permission to take some time for yourself. From my research on adolescent writing groups and staff nurses writing in groups, I know that writing can increase self esteem and self efficacy. Both esteem and efficacy you can loose fast in nursing school. A student reports:

It helps me to vent on paper, to just write out what is bothering me. To write out how crappy I feel, or write who I am mad at, to write how sad some patients make me feel, to write out all my frustrations. Journaling helps me. Sometime I need to dump it all on the page before I can talk to someone.

Writing can also inform you about how much you know. Consider that all the narratives in this book have been written by students about experiences that they have been carrying around with them. Keep a journal of your own thoughts and feelings. Document your experiences. Your words are precious.

Diversion

Some students say that they could not manage nursing school if they did not play a sport. Athletics provide a whole body diversion. Other students find relief going to work at a non–health care job. Amber writes:

I love my job as a swim instructor because it has nothing to do with nursing. It's nice to just escape for a little while.

In my student interviews, no student came right out and said it, but playing, having fun, and being silly is a key to your sanity. It is tricky to balance play and the work of learning to be a nurse, but it is possible and it is required. Remember my friend's study that I mentioned in an earlier chapter, when every time she went to interview an expert nurse, if they were not at work they were not in town! When the experts had time off they left town to go and play whether it be snowboarding, beach walking, hiking with good friends, or relaxing with family, their time away replenished them and contributed to them being able to be focused, yet balanced, when they were on the job.

Connections

Finding time to connect with others and finding time to be quiet by yourself can provide diversion, energy, and emotional support.

My friends help me manage stress. Some of us are better at not being stressed out than others. I find my friends who are good at it and spend time with them.

Sometimes I like to go visit friends at other schools. It helps to be away from your school for a little while and remember what fun feels like.

My friends are the most important thing to me. They make me laugh and laughing really keeps me sane. They make nursing school fun along the way. It's hard, but you're supposed to enjoy it too.

Significant relationships can provide support *or* can divert you from what you need to do.

Relationships are so important. If I didn't have my girlfriend I don't know what I would do. She helps to keep me calm when she tells me: it's okay to hate parts of it because you know that there are some parts that you love and you have come so far and worked so hard. When someone knows you really well, they see what you go through in school and can be that third party who looks in and reminds you how far you've come when you can't see it.

To many undergraduates, family provides critical support. Calling mom is part of the weekly routine.

I need my family. You learn to appreciate them when you go away to school, no matter what you're studying.

There's nothing better than going home to get away from it all for a little while. It helps to remember where you come from and all the people who are so proud of what you're doing.

Kick boxing, aerobics, or shooting hoops are good for the heart and the head. Meditation can provide the quiet rest you will need to balance school and life. Yoga, mindfulness meditation, tai chi, a massage, or walk in the woods can all provide you with the opportunity to stay grounded and get in touch with your own spirit. That is the spirit that got you into school in the first place and the spirit that is going to make you an awesome nurse. That part of you needs to be nurtured too. It does not work to run on empty for long. You know that.

SCHOOL AND FAMILY: JUGGLE OR BALANCE?

It is possible to have a family and go to school. It is not the easiest route but it is a road that many have traveled. I had my three children during my doctoral program. I started in September and my first child was born on November 12. Compared to my other years in school, my undergrad and Master's years, I was much more focused and actually more prepared in the PhD program. I had to be. When the kids were napping I was studying, before they got up, I was studying, after they went to bed, I was studying. It can work but both you and your family have to prepare.

When you are looking into school, look into child care, a house cleaner, backup support, and partner flexibility. If you were the mom or dad who did certain essential jobs at home, like grocery shopping, meal preparation, laundry, pick up, drop off, these tasks will need to be brought up for discussion and probably delegated. One faculty member tells students who are mothers: "Forget Thanksgiving. This year you are not going to be shopping, preparing, decorating, or serving. You will be writing a paper, studying for an exam, reading four pharmacology chapters, writing a thirty-page care plan." So make a care plan for you and your family so everyone understands what to expect and buys into the plan. This is your time. I have seen the most traditional woman come back to school and figure it out. You can do it too. Just plan ahead and don't pussyfoot around. Tell your 1-year-old to your senior in high school what to expect. Your family will be very proud of your tremendous accomplishment, so go for it!

NONTRADITIONAL STUDENTS IN A TRADITIONAL PROGRAM

Some students decide to return to school later, when their kids go to school, after the kids are raised or during a mid-career change. These students are older than 20, have life experience to add to their education, and, as Monica said, "We arrive at school with the baggage of our life." There may be a handful of older students or only one in a traditional baccalaureate class. There are more over-20-year-old students in a community college program. The nontraditional students insist becoming a nurse later in life is certainly possible, but there are unique circumstances that the more mature student needs to keep in mind. Susan relates:

My daughter was in the ER the night before my first day of classes. We were in the ER with her, worried, pacing, waiting until 6 A.M. At 9:00 I walked into my first nursing class.

Rose started her nursing career later in life, in a 2-year program:

When I was graduating from high school, most of my friends were heading off to college to become teachers or nurses. Me? I had no interest in it. Yes, I liked the medical field but in high school I followed the business courses—typing, shorthand, filing, etc. and I knew that I could find my place as a medical secretary. Years later as I sat there and typed about electrolytes and blood counts, the histories and physicals, the old flicker for nursing began to appear again. I once again began to think I could learn so much more and be more satisfied working as a nurse. One of the first things I had told my new boss was that I wanted to become a nurse. Her reaction? "Go for it!" My youngest child of three was in kindergarten when I started school. Again, I found myself taking care of everyone else, when they were quietly in bed, I would settle down, exhausted, to do my work.

Monica, going for her BS after her children were grown, admits:

You have sick kids, you juggle with your husband or bring them in with you for your exam.

Nontraditional students talk about school being a collective effort between your partner, the kids, and your extended family. It would be wise to bring everyone into the picture as soon as you are planning to return to school so you can get the family on board early. Students told me, "My daughter consoled me when I thought I could not understand the complicated text book." And, "I called my son at college when I have to write my first paper. Help! I called him back when I got an A!" Rose started in a community college program and returned for a baccalaureate degree later:

When my youngest went off to college in 2003, I started to think about my goals again. I joined the gym and looked into the RN-BSN program. I told myself that if my prerequisites were too involved, I would not do it. To my surprise, they looked pretty manageable. I again signed up for prerequisite classes at the community college. I found I still had the joy of learning, the only difference was not only was I older but I was downright OLD!

Remember, when you start out, this is the first nursing class for everyone, whether 20 years old or 50 years old. Look around. These are your peers. They look a lot like your kids. They live in the dorms, hang out with friends, bar-hop on Thirsty Thursdays, and are just as nervous as you are about doing well and surviving clinical. Many of your new, young colleagues have complicated lives as well. Their young age belies the adult issues they are dealing with. Undergraduates are handling grandparents being ill, parents dying, siblings having life problems, roommates being depressed, considering an abortion or dealing with an eating disorder in addition to the first time away from home, having a boyfriend/girlfriend or not having a boyfriend/girlfriend. They have interesting lives and study skills, they party too much or never go out, and they have the same goal as you: to become a nurse.

The older students tell me that to survive you have to befriend your younger peers. You have to become part of their study groups, part of their clinical rotation and part of their just hangin' out. Of course, you have no time for just hangin' out but you cannot get through the program alone. It is lonely enough being out of sync:

I feel like in every class I had this cloak of invisibility. You are totally ignored by the instructor. You consistently hear "when you grow up and learn a little more . . ." So it is up to me to reach out.

Florence Nightingale said the nursing student should be a mature, young woman. Our 20-year-olds recognize how difficult it is to be in college and study a very serious practice profession. There may never be a right time. I started my undergraduate program at 17. There was no question that I was way too immature. I went back to grad school on the younger side. At 24 years old, as I looked around the room I felt like I might not have enough experience to be in graduate school. In my PhD program, I was more pregnant than anyone in the room! There may never be a right time, but we know that older students bring a wealth of experience, knowledge of life, and a previous career to build on. Returning students make excellent nurses. So gather your support, plan out your coursework, connect to your new peer. There is no time like the present.

MENTORING: GOOD FOR BOTH PARTIES

It is helpful to have a mentor and it is rewarding to be a mentor. Students can really benefit from having an older student (just a class ahead will do) provide mentoring. Mentors are people who teach, guide, counsel, and coach. Ideally, the mentor and protégé find each other on their own. The mentor sees a younger person who she or he feels a connection to, see qualities they could develop, and a personality that compliments theirs. Protégés may find a person they admire and want to be like and invite the more senior person to be their mentor. Sounds good and works well on the job too. But in school you barely have time to make friends, let alone find a mentor, so it is better to be assigned to a more senior student who can answer questions about classes and clinicals, to help you to know what not to stress about and what is important to focus on. Some schools provide these connections, others will if students ask for them. My advice: ask for a mentor connection. An experienced student's advice: it is so worth it! There will be more on mentoring in Chapter 6.

CONCLUSION

This is a longer chapter because doing well in nursing school is no small task. Knowing the four stages of role transition will be useful to keep in mind. Listening to advice from those who have been there can give you a heads up on what is to come. The skills of organization, time management, and managing clinical are key to being successful in school. Managing stress is essential to your life as a student and to your lifelong career. Doing well in school as 20-year-old or 50-year-old is a reasonable goal well worth pursuing!

END-OF-CHAPTER EXERCISE: BEEN THERE, DONE THAT

You've been in school before, you know what works for you. You come with good experience you need to remember as you take this new task on. Let's think about what you bring to your studies:

1. What study skills have you already developed?

2. What sort of organizational skills do you already have?

3. What organizational skills can you build on? What new ones do you need to develop?

4. How have you budgeted your time?

5. How do you manage stress now?

6. What kind of stress strategies can you develop?

You have a base for school already. In your heart you know what works and what doesn't. Listen to that voice. Begin to prepare for this life-changing event now. I just had dinner with a group of graduating seniors. Everyone was thrilled about the jobs they already had been offered. Their salary ranged from $25 to $30 per hour. They were psyched! Keep that goal in mind.

References

Arrien, A. (1993). *The four fold way*. San Francisco, CA: HarperSanFrancisco.

Lamott, A. (1995). *Bird by bird*. New York: Anchor Books.

[CHAPTER 6]

Moving On!

The Transition from Student to Nurse

After 4 years of nursing school, students are ready to leave behind 20-page care plans, reflective clinical journals, and computerized exams. Students are anxious to transition into practice and see a paycheck!

A transition is defined as the passage from one stage to another. Recent graduates report that, although nursing students have been out in the field since their first nursing course, moving into a job still feels like a giant leap into the unknown rather than the planned, smooth approach that the word transition implies. Bridges (1980) describes a state of transition as a time of uncertainty, when the past is receding rapidly but the future has not yet arrived.

That's it! You are ready to leave but you do not know where you are going. That in-between phase is when people are most vulnerable. So if you are feeling chaotic, confused, and stressed, you are right where you should be, leaving the past behind but your future has not yet arrived. This is a time to talk to faculty mentors who can give you some insight into your experience. This is the time to talk to nurses who have recently gone through the transition. That is exactly what we are going to do in this chapter, hear from new nurses who have been there.

Although nurses insist they are the hardest working students on campus, they still experience the reality shock of the work world. Working nights, working on holidays, taking care of patients all . . . on . . . your . . . own, is still a shock. In this chapter, we will take a close look at moving into the novice nurse role from applying for jobs to orientation, by listening to new nurses who have made the transition from school to work.

We will learn about the five essential components that can buffer the shock and facilitate a successful transition:

1. A solid support network
2. A substantial orientation
3. A caring nurse manager
4. A preceptor that fits
5. A mentor that matches

But first, let's listen to the experience of a few recent graduates. I knew Alena since freshman year in the Introduction to Nursing course. She was highly motivated, always prepared for clinical, actively participated in class, and did well on exams. There was no question she would make a fine nurse. Here Alena tells us about her so-called transition into practice:

During my (student) internship in my last semester of school in a "Transition" lecture my teacher said, "I graduated from nursing school knowing everything, and got to my first job knowing nothing." Alena reports, "That has been my experience on the floor thus far." On my first day, I kept saying to myself, "I am a nurse, I am a nurse." The truth was I felt nothing like a nurse, a graduate, or a person who had studied ridiculously hard for the past five years. I felt like a person who came off the street, wandered into the hospital, and was told to go take a blood sugar.

Now that is a reality description of taking the leap. The transition period is an adventure even for the best of students. Recall the four stages of role transition in Chapter 4: honeymoon, shock, acceptance, and resolution. As a novice nurse, Alena, in the first month of employment, was in the shock stage. The five components of a successful transition were developed from Alena's experience and other real students who have made the leap into practice. You need to keep in mind, though you are an experienced student you are still a novice nurse. Go easy on yourself.

THE NEW NURSE

Patricia Benner (1984) studied how practicing nurses progress from being a novice to an expert. From her research, she identified five stages of role development:

1. Novice

2. Advanced beginner

3. Competent

4. Proficient

5. Expert

Without nursing experience to draw on, the novice nurse only has the rules, procedures, and policies to follow. Procedures are important but a list of rules does not assist the nurse in interpreting the subtleties of each individual patient situation. Yet, the lack of experience coupled with the fact that every new nurse student is afraid they will make a mistake and kill someone, forces the new nurse to rely on all they have, that is, rules. I recall one student, Maria, telling me about her first abdominal dressing change. Maria described rehearsing sterile technique in the back room, gathering all the necessary equipment, rehearsing sterile technique one more time outside the patient's room before she went in and set up the equipment on the patient's bedside table. Next, Maria called in her instructor to observe her meticulously perform a dressing change. As she applied the last piece of tape, she heard her instructor quietly say, "Good job." Maria breathed a sigh of relief, looked up, and noticed that the patient had a head. She looked at the patient for the first time and realized she was so focused on getting the procedure right, following the rules to a tee, that she forgot to say a word to the patient. Maria admitted that she was successful in performing the dressing change but had a lot to learn about giving patient care.

Dee, a new nurse, gives us a very honest account of her awareness of a task-focus approach. Dee recognizes that without experience, rules are all she has to go on:

As a new nurse I understand I am very task oriented, because I want to be efficient with my time. I make a list of things that need to be done and I check them off as I go: flow sheet, morning meds, check blood sugar, hang IV med, write nursing note. Because I'm still working on efficiency, I'm not good at anticipating my patients' needs. For example, I had a confused, noncompliant, and very anxious patient that was going to be discharged to a nursing home at 1 P.M. My patient had Ativan ordered as a PRN med for anxiety and if I were thinking ahead I would have given him a dose at 12 P.M. so that he would've been relatively calm by the time the ambulance came to transfer him. When the ambulance arrived all of his paperwork was ready and I had called report to the facility that was accepting him but when it was time for him to move it took the EMTs 20 minutes to calm him down and get him on the stretcher. When the nurse asked me why I hadn't given him a sedative I couldn't tell her it wasn't on my list of things to do, so I apologized and admitted I hadn't thought of it. I've been told that anticipating clients' needs will come in time but it didn't keep me from feeling pretty foolish that day.

Dee is the picture of a novice nurse, doing what she should be doing: focusing on organizing, prioritizing, and task accomplishment. Dee is gaining experience one patient at a time. Alena watched the skill of expert nurses unfold before her novice eyes:

My first patient came to the floor: a triple A repair with hypertension, a doctor quickly following him. "He has a trauma line . . . be careful," the resident said directly to me. I lifted up my hands, pointed to my preceptor and said, "That's the nurse." I didn't want to be rude but I didn't want the resident thinking that I could do anything with the information he had given me. I stood para-lyzed, watching the resident run through orders and what they had done in the OR. The nurses seemed to absorb the information effortlessly while they hooked the patient up to a cardiac monitor, did an EKG, set up a CVP trans-ducer, and watched the steadily increasing arterial blood pressure. "Did you prescribe something to bring that down?" the nurse calmly asked. "Ya I did, you can also set up the fentanyl drip."

"Put this on low intermittent," said a nurse as she handed me the end of this gentleman's NG tube. I guess she noted my deer-in-headlights reaction and gave me directions to where the suction tubing was located. This is how my day started.

Alena's description is a perfect example of why it is critical for novice nurses to have experienced, approachable nurses to work with. In a study of novice nurses and adverse events (Ebright & Urdan, 2004), the researchers reported that the current health care environment of under-staffing, overwork, and use of per diem nurses not only jeopardizes patient care but also hinders the development of the new nurse. As you interview for jobs, it is important to notice the staffing, the team functioning (or not), and the amount of per diem staff. Staffing, workload expectations, senior staff availability, and the use of auxiliary nurses will affect the quality of your job from orientation to functioning independently.

The nurse who is an *advanced beginner* has a little more experience than the novice. They begin to recognize global aspects of situations that have been pointed out by their preceptor or that they have picked up from caring for similar types of patients.

The *competent* nurse has worked with similar patients for a year or two and knows the common trajectory of illness, the possible outcomes, and the discharge expectations. The *proficient* nurse is flexible, able to anticipate normal responses, and recognizes patient nuances that indicate they do not fit within the expected critical path. The *expert* nurse has the depth of experience so they do not rely on rules but, rather, intuitively knows what is relevant in the situation. Their intuition has developed from years of experience and a deep understanding of the total situation. Before your start on the path to becoming an expert nurse, we need to recognize that the transition to a nurse begins in the first nursing course where you hear about the requirement for procuring a license before you can practice as a nurse.

NATIONAL COUNSEL LICENSING EXAM: NCLEX

To work in any state as a registered nurse, after you graduate, you will need to pass the licensing exam, the National Counsel Licensing Exam-for Registered Nurses, affectionately known as NCLEX. The exam tests for minimum nursing competence. You will hear about the NCLEX exam from the first day of your school orientation to the last day of classes. Most classes are designed to prepare you to successfully pass the exam by developing critical thinking skills, test-taking strategies, and familiarity with the content and format of the exam. Many teachers require an NCLEX review book to go with their course so that students can practice answering questions as they learn the course content. There are several comprehensive review books, CDs, and review courses available (see Appendix B at the end of the book). There is a lot to learn in school. The best advice is to look over the review books and purchase one as soon as you are accepted into the program. This book will become your new best friend. You will be spending a lot of time together. In addition, many programs have course-specific computer-assisted instruction and computerized exam packets that are designed to measure the student's ability to apply nursing knowledge to clinical practice. Several studies indicate success on the computerized exams predicts success on the NCLEX (Nibert, Young, & Adamson, 2006; Nibert & Young, 2006; Laucher, Newman, & Britt, 2006). Studying for the licensing exam in every course will increase both the competence and confidence needed to successfully pass the licensing exam. After graduation there are many independent review courses to choose from.

REVIEW COURSES

Many schools offer postgraduate access to test-taking strategies, use of the computer lab, planned review sessions, and an opportunity to join a study group. A review course separate from your program can also be very helpful. Just make sure the review course incorporates test-taking tips and test anxiety strategies. Some health care organizations offer NCLEX review courses for their new hires (this is a good question to ask on your interview). Take advantage of every exam preparation opportunity, within reason, that is. Two students just reported that they paid good money to take two review courses and after the exam they felt that they could have passed without either course. Now, these students are self-starters who have studied all along and religiously practiced review questions. Other students have enough work keeping up in school so that they do not start preparing for the exam until after graduation. You will have time after graduation to study if you create a daily routine where you take practice tests, use the computerized tests to get used to the style of the exam, and review areas of nursing that you have identified. All of the test books have review sections on each area of nursing. Review what you know and review what you do not know. Two recent graduates reported that they took a 3-week trip to Europe between graduation and the NCLEX exam. They practiced a few questions on Eurorail but basically relaxed, came home, and successfully passed the test.

You have to decide what will assist you in preparing for the exam. Appendix B, at the end of the book, is a list of some NCLEX preparation resources.

PASS, NO PASS

The results of a study (Firth, Sewell, & Clark, 2006) of students who passed the NCLEX and students who did not pass revealed that the students who passed took responsibility for their learning, prepared over time, when they felt ready they took the exam, and they were comfortable using stress management strategies before and during the exam. Students who did not pass the exam on the first try reported that they had not developed a study plan that fit their needs, they were not prepared for the format of the exam, they did not feel able to manage the critical thinking aspects of the exam, and they were unable to manage their test anxiety. So here is what's important:

1. Developing a study routine that fits your learning style (which still means studying every day)
2. Study on your own and with others
3. Use a book, a CD *and* a computerized test
4. Find a review course that fits your time frame and your budget
5. Take advantage of the support your school offers. They want you to be successful!
6. Learn stress management skills that work for you. Stress management takes practice, start to employ stress strategies into your daily routine as soon as possible.

Whether you pass the first time or not does not dictate the kind of nurse you will be. John, my graduate teaching assistant, reminded all undergraduates that the NCLEX is a door you need to pass through to become a nurse, so don't let that door get in your way to the career you have studied for. Neusa, a top student and a leader on campus, reports:

The worst feeling is when you fail the NCLEX and already have a job position waiting for you. You were a good student in nursing school, spent months studying and you still did not make it. This is exactly what happened to me. I am not sure what I did wrong the first time around. I had studied hard for this test, took advantage of taking the Kaplan course in my last semester then took a review course after graduation. I thought I was prepared.

It was a sunny afternoon when I took the to train to the testing center. I was not nervous when I first got there but I began feel the beads of sweat on my forehead as I started to read the questions and was not sure about my answers. My heart was racing as I told myself to take deep breaths. I spent 4 grueling hours taking the test. After moving through 250 questions all I wanted is for the computer to shut down. I couldn't think any longer. Everything looked dark from my point of view. I came home crying knowing that I did a terrible job on the test. What was my weakness preparing for the test? To this day I am not sure. However, the support and motivation I received from my family, friends, former professors, nursing recruiter, and manager was crucial. I still had my position available at the hospital and the nursing recruiter was very supportive. She said, "Neusa, don't worry about it, I am sure you will pass it next time, many people don't pass it their first time. You still have a job with us, but let me know if you need any help." I was so relieved when I heard these words. All I needed was some time to relax and begin studying again. For a week I did not study and the following week I signed up to retake the NCLEX course. I learned to read more carefully into the questions so I could choose the correct answer. When English is not your first language this test is even more challenging. You may interpret the question wrong which may lead you to choose a wrong answer.

When I took the test for the second time I passed it right away, I only had 75 questions. I knew I had passed it this time; there was an internal feeling that told me. I went shopping to celebrate, even though I did not have the results yet, I was so sure that I did a great job and I was right!

I believe it is important for students to know that it is okay if you do not pass the NCLEX the first time. That doesn't demonstrate how much you know or how good of a nurse you can be. It is important not to give up, but make the best out of every situation. Nothing can stop you except your own self.

The bottom line is, the exam is a challenge for everyone. Take the study tips seriously, practice, practice, practice, and work on your own test stress plan. Three months after Neusa passed the exam, she went on to receive the Excellence in Nursing award. See the Children's Hospital web site to learn more about recognition awards. http://www.childrenshospital. org/chnews/03–01–07/nursing_excellence_times_four.html

Once you have passed the exam, you can start to work. Some facilities will not even consider new applicants until after they have passed the licensing exam. Other places welcome your interest and encourage you to send an application in advance. Each facility and each geographic area has its hiring windows. Once you have determined the region that you want to work in, find out when hiring begins so you can plan your life between graduation and job interviews. The search for a job usually begins at least 6 months before graduation. Some places are looking to interview new graduates fall semester senior year. *Do not* wait for your school to direct you, identify the facilities that you are interested in, and find out when they start to interview. About half of the senior nursing students accept a position before graduation. The other half decide to wait until after their licensing exam and a well-deserved vacation. Fortunately, in this era of a shortage of nurses, there will be jobs looking for nurses no matter when you decide to begin your search.

JOB SEARCH

Whether you realize it or not, from your first clinical rotation you will be looking around at job possibilities. You will have the opportunity to observe nurses, care for patients, and collaborate with the health care team. While working in clinical rotations, you will see nurses you want to be like and some that do not fit your ideal. There will be role models and mentors that you will meet as you progress through your program. Keep your mind open. Most students start their nursing education with an idea about what type of nurse they would like to be. In fact, the majority of freshmen see themselves working in labor and delivery or in pediatrics. The babies and the kids. That makes sense. Yet, listen to this, in my last clinical, where the juniors rotate through pediatrics, maternity, and psychiatry, all eight students did not like maternity or pediatrics but loved psychiatry. Who would guess? So keep your eyes and ears open. Try to notice the difference between the units that you rotate through:

- Which floors feel supportive?
- Where are the nurses happy?
- Where is there a sense of team collaboration?

One recent graduate reported that she was placed in her ideal internship in an intensive care unit. But as Kavita worked in her internship with patients that were so critically ill, she noticed that 10 out of 12 of the patients probably would not make it. She decided as a new nurse this was too sad to deal with every day. She needed to take care of patients who would get well and leave the hospital. She is now satisfied in her first job on a general medical-surgical unit. A general unit can be a good place to start out but is not required. Starting on a general unit gives you an opportunity to get your skills down and build your knowledge base. You have plenty of time to specialize. Like Kavita, you need to decide what works for you.

As you think about your professional and personal aspirations consider whether a large teaching acute care setting or smaller community hospital would meet your needs. Will it make a difference to work in a Magnet facility? Some hospitals have been awarded the distinction of Magnet status from the American Nurses' Credentialing Center (ANCC), an affiliate of the American Nurses Association. Basically, Magnet means that because of the programs, support, recognition of nurses as well as the excellent patient outcomes achieved, nurses report high job satisfaction and low job turnover. The 14 forces of magnetism are outlined on the

ANCC site (http://www.nursecredentialing.org/magnet/). So you have a well-rounded perspective of the effect of magnet status, consider the diverse opinions about magnet status. Some of the concerns are outlined by the Center for Nurse Advocacy. The mission of the center is to facilitate understanding of the central role of nursing in health care; check out the site at http://www.nursingadvocacy.org. To assist you in assessing job possibilities, check out the web sites listed in Appendix C at the end of the book and consider meeting with career services.

CAREER SERVICES

By senior year, you will have a better idea where you might want to work and if you have an internship in our final semester that experience will add to your fact-finding. You can begin the job search by updating your résumé and consulting with career services. Depending on the capacity of your school's career services office you may have access to career counseling, career job fairs, résumé workshops, and internship possibilities. Many schools have excellent career counselors who are there to assist you in finding a job that fits your interests and in a location that fits your lifestyle. Career fairs are when hospitals come to your school or to a central location to set up booths with information about their facilities and hand out marketing materials designed to let you know what the nursing positions are like and the opportunities for job progression in their organization. Many facilities offer opportunities to showcase their nursing department through new grad networking nights or new grad luncheons. Look at the web sites of facilities you want to learn more about to learn when they will be hosting new grads. Taking the opportunity to talk to nurses who work in the organization you are looking into or locating alums from your school that work in the type of setting you would like to work can be very helpful in narrowing your job search.

Career services usually offer workshops in résumé writing or they set up individual appointments with students. The next section takes you through what a career workshop offers.

PREPARING A RÉSUMÉ

Résumés are a summary of your education and experience. If you do not have much of experience, that is okay. What counts is that your résumé is a truthful, clear, and a succinct document. What should you include? It depends what position you are applying for. Read on.

You will have at least two résumés, one that stays on your computer and one that is designed to fit the job or education you are applying for. There is no generic résumé for all. Each time you send out a résumé, the content is designed to address the position that you want.

The computer résumé is where you store your experience or honors you receive, so you do not forget to include these items in your "going-out-the-door" résumé. For the résumé you send out include the following:

- The top 5 inches is the most important space on your résumé. You may want to put a one line "objective" right under your name and address so that the reader can see exactly what you are interested in. Make sure your e-mail address is professional, *not* Jennyhotlegs.com. Create a professional sounding voice mail on your phone as well.

- The résumé is a simple document designed to show content quickly. Make sure you capitalize, bold, or put a period in the same places for each line. This usually takes several edits to catch any thing that is not in place.

- Use reverse chronological order—under each new heading, the first entry is the most recent, and every entry after that gets older and older. Stay with a "book" font like Times New Roman, between 10–14 points. Don't get fancy with your résumé. This is a business document.

- Start with education. Your education will be the most significant and the first piece of information in your résumé. If you are right out of high school include special courses, class projects, community service learning, and large research papers that you are proud of. Include your GPA and SAT scores. I like when the dates of your education and experience are lined up in a column on the right or left hand side. That way I can find the dates easily. See the sample résumé in this chapter.

- Following education comes experience. Experience is experience, whether paid or unpaid, in the classroom or out. Experience should also be written in reverse chronological order. Under experience describe what you did (accomplishments, results, outcomes), not what you were supposed to do (responsibilities), and quantify what you did (numbers, percentages) as much as possible. Consider listing out relevent clinical experiance that you have accumulated while in school.

- You do not need to use pronouns (I, we, me, etc.) or articles (a, an, the). Stay away from *underlines* or *italics*—they do not scan or reproduce well. Stay away from résumé templates—everyone recognizes them and you look as though you do not care (so why should they?).
- Do use active and descriptive verbs.
- Use Microsoft Word so that everyone can open your file.
- Proofread, proofread, proofread. Human resource professionals say that typos and bad grammar are the very first reason résumés get thrown out.

There are whole sections in bookstores on writing résumés and many web sites that cover the details. Look around, have someone else proofread, print on plain white paper or be ready to attach to an e-mail in a Word document. Do not send anything that cannot be opened, like an RTF file or an Office Works file.

The résumé shown in Figure 6-1 is a model résumé. Do not hesitate to follow the format so you have an updated résumé to attach with online applications and you have a clean résumé to bring with you to your interview. When you mail your résumé send along a cover letter.

COVER LETTERS

I am a big fan of cover letters. This is your chance to be creative, upbeat, and enthusiastic. This is also a formal business letter, so follow *business letter guidelines.* First, make sure you have the correct name of the person you are sending the letter to. Start by telling them what position you are applying for. For example, Catherine wrote:

I am writing to express my interest in the staff nurse position on Ellison 16. I have chosen to apply to XXX because of its superior reputation as a teaching hospital and its excellence in patient care and research.

Sharon wrote:

I am seeking a registered nurse position on the medical–surgical unit at XXX Medical Center. My educational experience has provided me with an in-depth exposure to and exceptional knowledge of assessments and treatments of clients with various health disruptions.

Sally Street

837 Pine Street   413- 898-4354
Amherst, MA 01002   Sstreet@yahoo.com

Career Objective: to assume a staff nurse position on a medical unit

EDUCATION
University of Massachusetts Amherst, School of Nursing
  Bachelor of Science in Nursing   May 2006
  Commonwealth Honors Program

Springfield Technical Community College
  Associate in Nursing   May 2001

CLINICAL ROTATIONS
Baystate Medical Center, Springfield MA   Advanced senior practicum in
                                                                      Medicine/HIV+
Holyoke Hospital, Holyoke MA   Senior HIV/AIDS case study Marks
Meadow Elementary School, Amherst MA   Community Health
Western Massachusetts Hospital, Westfield MA   Pediatrics
Mary Lane Hospital, Ware MA   Medical/Surgical and Cardiac
University of Massachusetts Medical Center,
Worcester MA   Psychiatric/Mental Health

ASSOCIATION MEMBERSHIPS
National Student Nurses' Association
University of Massachusetts Amherst Student Nurses' Association

EXPERIENCE
Farren Care Center, Turners Falls, MA   2004 to present
Nurse's Aide—Provided rehabilitative nursing care to promote
and restore independence on both spinal cord and head trauma units.
Experience with ventilator dependent individuals, straight catherization,
bowel programs, tube feedings, dressing changes, tracheotomy and
colostomy care.

The Atrium at Cardinal Drive, Agawam, MA   2001–2002
Nurses' Aide—Provided complete evening care on skilled nursing unit.

Jerry Lewis Muscular Dystrophy Camp, Butler, PA   Summer 1999
Camp Counselor—Counseled child with Muscular Dystrophy.
Assisted campers with ADL's and encouraged participation in
planned events.

Figure 6-1. A résumé prepared by a recent graduate of a Bachelor's program in nursing.

LEADERSHIP EXPERIENCE

Alpha Chi Omega Sorority, Amherst, MA   2002–present
Community Service Chair—Organized and participated in activities
ranging from tutoring children at several local community centers
to playing bingo with residents of nursing home.

Habitat for Humanity, Alternate Spring Break   2004–present
Fund-raising Chair

Sophomore Representative to Clinical Faculty   2003–2004
Served as liaison between students and clinical faculty.

LANGUAGES
Fluent French, intermediate Hebrew, basic Spanish

Figure 6-1. (Continued)

Always have two paragraphs in your letter. The second paragraph may say
something more about you. From Catherine's letter, after describing the
position, she writes:

*As a second Bachelor's nursing student I believe I have a unique background
of professional, educational, and personal experiences that will make me a
positive addition to your health care team. These experiences, which are
detailed in my résumé, have strengthened my organizational skills and ability to prioritize, to develop my interpersonal and communication skills, to perform multiple task simultaneously, and to gain an appreciation of cultural
diversity.*

Kaye, who first tells the reader she is applying for a position in the child
birth center, then writes:

*I enjoyed my maternal-newborn rotation the most. I felt privileged to be able
to be a part of the beginning of life, witnessing the joy and pain of childbirth
while providing essential care and comfort. There is no word I can think of to
adequately describe the wondrous feeling of holding a newborn. It is these feelings that make maternal-newborn nursing so appealing to me.*

With these statements in the cover letter, I'd be very interested in
meeting these job applicants, wouldn't you? Finish up the letter by thank-
ing the reader for their consideration, saying you welcome the opportunity

to learn more about the position and you are looking forward to the interview. But use your own style to communicate these sentiments.

One last bit of advice: I am sure you have heard that you should also clean up your FaceBook pages. Think of what you'd want the nurse recruiter to see. You get the picture, so make sure your pictures look good. Now for the interview.

INTERVIEW

The preparation for a job interview is similar to the school interview in Chapter 4. When you are considering where to work you will want to go to the agency's web site and find out what the hospital's mission is, what the philosophy of the nursing department is, what is the nursing department's mission and vision? You will want to be able to speak to how you fit with the philosophy, mission, and vision and why you think you would be a good addition to their team. You will want to think through the categories of:

- Why do you want to be a nurse on this unit?
- How has your school program prepared you to work on this unit?
- What types of patients have you cared for that fits with our unit?
- Think of a stressful situation and how you handled it.

The following questions prompt you to develop answers that will be useful for your interview. You will want to be ready with stories that can illustrate your experience with being a:

- Patient advocate.
- Aware of patient safety.
- Being able to delegate.
- Demonstrate your awareness of common procedures used in the area of practice, common medications, and common treatments.
- Provide an example of thinking:
  - critical thinking
  - thinking on your feet
  - reflective practice
- Demonstrating collaboration on the health care team.

- Provide examples of how you have exhibited leadership (review Chapter 4 leadership principles).
- Demonstrate your interest in being involved in the organization:
    - What school committees were you on?
    - What community service projects were you involved in?
    - How have you already served as a mentor?
    - What nursing organizations do you belong to?
    - What nursing journals do you read?
    - Are you considering going on for more education?
- Indicate your awareness of the larger health environment and global concerns as you talk about your school and previous job experience.

In some interviews, you will be given patient scenarios and asked how you would respond or prioritize or delegate in the situation. Prepare for behavioral responses by reviewing NCLEX scenarios on communicating, prioritizing, and delegating. See Appendix B at the end of the book for a list of NCLEX study resources.

Reflection 1: Interview Preparation

Do not expect to spontaneously come up with exemplars of the topics listed above. That would be difficult for anyone. Prepare for the interview ahead of time by writing out your responses to each of the categories listed. Think of stories to illustrate each topic. Being prepared will decrease your interview anxiety markedly. When you have developed your own unique responses to the questions that will be asked consider role-playing an interview with a friend. During the interview, you may have to insert a few stories if you are not asked directly. Remember that few interviewers are trained in the process of interviewing so they may not know to ask certain questions. This means that you may have to stop them so you can tell them about yourself. I can guarantee following the interview you will be compared to other candidates that came in and you will stand out because you had stories to fit every question.

In preparation for the interview, you will also want to develop a list of questions in advance. Now this may seem preposterous for you, the newbie, to quiz your potential employer, but how else are you going to find out if this is the right place to start your career? Asking about the typical workload, the staffing on the unit, the use of per diem nurses, and the expectation of overtime will be important questions. A tour of the unit is essential to give you a feel for the work environment. A question and answer opportunity with staff can be enormously helpful. To take advantage of talking to senior staff consider how you will handle yourself, the questions you will ask and the responses you will give, prior to the interview. This job is what you have been studying for, dreaming about and counting down the days until you could begin. The organization invests time and money into recruiting and retaining new nurses. And this is your first job as a nurse. Both you and your employer want to make sure this is a good fit.

Review the information at http://www.aacn.nche.edu, "What Every Nursing Graduate Should Consider When Seeking Employment."

DRESS REHEARSAL

Practice, practice, practice before you go to any interview. A dress rehearsal is essential. You may not notice the influence of practicing until you are in the interview, but trust me, with practice you will feel prepared. Start with planning ahead for what you will say when you first walk in, what you will wear, and what you will bring with you on the interview; hint: a clean résumé, a notepad, a pen, and a sheet with references. Before the interview, on the notepad you might want to jot down key words to the stories you want to share so in the midst of wanting to do well in the interview you can recall what you had planned to say. You may also want to write out the questions that you want answers to.

Reflection 2: Lights, Cameras, and You're On!

Start your rehearsal by envisioning walking into the interview. Take a moment, close your eyes, take a deep breath, and see yourself walking into the interview.

• What do you say?

• What do you do?

• Will you shake the secretary's hand?

• Introduce yourself, first and last name?

Your interview starts with your e-mails and phone calls with the secretary. Your in-person meeting begins at the front desk. Plan what you will say. Remember that secretaries have a lot of influence. In my role as a manager, after the candidate left the interview, I would walk out and ask my assistant what he thought. He has seen a lot of people come and go. I valued his input and so should you!

Plan on what you are going to wear well in advance. Try your whole interview outfit on *before* the night before. Then, just like your first day of elementary school, lay your interview clothes out the night before so you do not have to hunt for polished shoes or a clean pair of socks. Business conservative is the look you are going for. CONSERVATIVE deserves capital letters. Once you feel comfortable with your interview look, decide what you will bring with you.

Prepare what you will bring with you ahead of time:

1. Directions to the facility
2. Parking information
3. Phone number of the interviewer
4. Directions to the office
5. A clean résumé
6. A notebook
7. A smile and a warm handshake
8. *Do not* bring a cup of coffee with you

Think of one of your role models. How would they handle an interview? Think about how you want to be perceived. Then make it happen!

Once you have had the interview send a brief thank you note within twenty-four hours. If you have conducted the whole application process online, then send a thank you e-mail. This is one more chance to let them know you are the best choice for the job!

A SOLID SUPPORT NETWORK

This transition stage is an adventure for every new nurse. Now that you are leaving all your school support behind you will need to think about developing an expanded support network.

Reflection 3: Your Support Network

Social support is the key to growth. At times we need instrumental support which can be actual hands on help or financial support and other times we need emotional support, like encouragement and connection. Who are the people that provide you with support? In a recent class, students reported that actually mapping out their support network was very informative. They could see who they needed to be in touch with and where they needed to expand their network. To describe your support network draw a diagram of "mind map" and consider the following questions:

1. Draw a circle in the center of the page and put your name in the middle.

2. Draw rays out from the circle.

3. At the end of the rays on one side of the circle, put your personal supports, on the other side of the circle write down your professional supports. Now ask yourself the following questions:

- Who nurtures you, lets you know your unique qualities?
- Who challenges you to reach and grow as a person?
- Who do you have fun with, relax, and laugh with?
- Who do you go to talk about difficult issues, vent anger, get feedback?
- Who would you lend money or let borrow your car?
- Who gives you career advice, encouragement, and support?

- Who has been with you while you have been thrilled to the top and down in the dumps while learning to be a nurse?
- Who do you go to for professional advice, to get support for your decisions?

See Figure 4-1 for an example of a mind map.

Questions: Look over your support network and consider:

1. Does your network need to be broadened? Are there other people you need to be in contact with?

2. Does your support network need more depth? Do you need to catch up with some of the individuals in your personal and professional support network to let them know what you are up to?

October reflects back on the support necessary to practice as a nurse:

I realized that a nurse is not just an individual but also a part of a group. It was the support from the group: doctors, other nurses, and support staff that allowed me to come into my own and supported the patient care that I was proud of.

In our society we often focus on the individual, look at the world as how it affects us individually. We choose to hold our breath in and keep life out. By taking a deep breath, I was able to connect with something bigger than myself. It is that faith in something larger than me that has helped me survive and thrive in what can be a challenging field. Without the people who provided support and confidence along the way, I would not be who I am today, a nurse.

New jobs are challenging. Both personal and professional support are necessary to feel like you can take on this new role. Your orientation should be designed to provide you with the professional support you need to begin the job.

A SUBSTANTIAL ORIENTATION

Alena passed the licensing test, drove across country, and dove into her new job:

I took the boards in Springfield in July . . . and passed! I went home to NY for a week and then took a 6-day road trip to Portland Oregon. Within the first week of being I got a nursing job at Oregon Health and Science University Hospital in Portland. October 9th I started their 10-week critical care internship. I am taking classes, doing homework, and doing two-day shifts a week with a preceptor. It's basically nursing school all over except I'm getting paid. I am working in the cardiac surgical intensive care unit. I'll start for real when I complete the program in December and then I'll be on nights.

Alena points out two critical aspects of every new job that can facilitate a successful transition: a substantial orientation and a good preceptor. A 6-week to 3-month orientation can develop a solid base to work from. A preceptor that is a competent, approachable nurse that you feel comfortable with is the key. Amanda describes her first weeks:

My first shift on orientation as an official registered nurse was an 11 P.M.– 7 A.M. shift. I arrived 45 minutes early and sat in my car with a large cup of Dunkin Donuts coffee absolutely freaking out, not only because tonight I would begin my career, but also because never, not even in the peak of final exams, had I ever stayed up all night long.

By the time I arrived on the floor I had a pretty good caffeine buzz going on so I was feeling especially bubbly when I ran into a group of CNAs who were taking a break. "Hi! I'm Amanda! I'm a new nurse!" I said enthusiastically.

"Oh yeah, we've been waiting to see the new orientee," one girl replied.

"Uh, yup! See you around!"

Eventually, I found my preceptor and she quickly ran through a bunch of logistical things. She gave me the list of our patients and we went through the patient kardex together. She was talking so fast and telling me a lot of things that I would need to commit to memory, and all I wished was that I could have a larger piece of paper to write all of it down on. We then checked on the patients. That was when I started to get nervous. The unit was a pediatric respiratory unit. Most of the patients were kids on ventilators. When I was shown how to take a child off a ventilator to suction her trache, ambu her in between suctioning, and maintain sterile technique all at the same time I thought I was doomed and that whenever I had to do this by myself, someone was going to end up dead. (To be continued)

Neusa went right to a specialty unit and was placed in the 5.5-month expanded orientation for new graduates to support her growth as a nurse:

As a novice nurse at Children's Hospital, Boston, Bone Marrow transplant unit I was accepted to be a part of a 22 weeks program offered to their new graduates. It is a fairly new program, which is making my transition from student to nurse very smooth. The staff understands that as a new graduate one needs practice, familiarity, and hands-on experience in order to feel comfortable and become a proficient nurse.

I love the fact that the program is divided into sessions which allow us, new graduates, to not panic, but continue to work gradually until we begin to feel comfortable with our role. The first session is 8 weeks long and its focus is academic. The second session is also 8 weeks long, but it's clinically based. The third or final session is 6 weeks long and I will be learning about crisis resource management and professional advancement at Children's Hospital, Boston. Currently I am taking academic courses, I am also working closely with my preceptor and the staff development faculty to manage patient care.

Following orientation, many places offer monthly new grad groups. You will always be too busy to attend these groups but you will also lose out on peer networking if you do not make time to attend. Recently, Jodi, a new nurse, told us how essential the new grad meetings were:

In the new grad group they ask you things that you need to talk about, that you need to hear from other new grads about, like

- *Are you taking care of yourself?*
- *Do you get off the floor for lunch?*
- *When was your first big error?*
- *What is it like to work on holidays?*

Without a peer group of new grads, you may become disillusioned from the combination of being new, having to learn so much, and leaving behind your old school support network. Disillusionment can precipitate isolation and self-doubt. When these feelings arise, as they will, recognize this is a stage that you can predict and that you need to go through. To maintain your sanity, you need to be talking to your preceptor and other new nurses. You need to go through this stage with other new nurses. Remember sophomore/junior year when you went through the negative stage, questioning assignments, faculty, and clinical nurses? Remember the disillusion with your program and your career choice? In school, it was easier to rally other students to the cause. The same thing, feeling disillusioned and disenchanted, happens in a new job. It just might take a little more to find peers to share your concerns with. But that is exactly what you need to do. Keep in touch with your school friends. Melissa recognizes how helpful peers can be:

It has also been helpful that I have kept in touch with many other UMass grads via e-mail as we all start our new careers and lives. I always know that whatever I am going through, that all my friends are experiencing the same things! It's very comforting.

Every new grad emphasized the importance of a solid, self-paced orientation, a good preceptor match, and a management team that was supportive of new grads.

A CARING NURSE MANAGER

For new nurses, the manager feels way above them. However, we know from research that the manager has a tremendous impact on the staff nurse's daily work life. In Tucker and Edmundson's (2002) study on nurse problem solving, they found that nurses were more likely to address problems that came up when the manger was present, accessible, and they were known for following through on issues that staff bring up. So when you are interviewing for jobs, it is important to pay attention to how you feel with the nurse manager; notice how they relate to you and notice how they relate to their staff. Kavita, a recent graduate, reported that the managers would check in with her every couple of weeks to make sure things were going well for her. From the beginning, she felt support from the top down. Her preceptor was another person she could count on.

A PRECEPTOR MATCH

Preceptors and the staff development office are key resources for the new nurse. A preceptor is a more senior nurse assigned to a new nurse for a certain time period, usually from 6 months to a year. The nurse manager will match an orientee with a staff nurse preceptor. The preceptor generally serves as a touchstone for the new nurse. The orientee may begin by shadowing the preceptor before they are assigned their own patients. The preceptor is there to guide the new nurse in learning unit routines, clinical procedures, communication channels, and the organizational culture. The culture of the unit is the unwritten rules that have evolved overtime, such as the interaction during shift hand-off, how the break schedule is managed, the typical lunch routine, or the relationships with other departments. The preceptor will guide the new nurse through the shift offering advice and role modeling. The preceptor role differs in every organization. One new grad was assigned a primary preceptor and also had a secondary, backup preceptor as she rotated shifts.

Although the nurse manager is very interested in making the transition smooth for the new nurse, sometimes the preceptor/orientee match does not connect. In that case, the new nurse should consult with the manager. Two new graduates from two different institutions talked about their first preceptor not working out. Both nurses took the initiative to meet with their manager and felt supported in their perceptions. As a result, a change in preceptor was judiciously arranged. More formal education for orientees comes through the staff development office.

The staff development office provides internal educational opportunities for every level of nurse. Staff development may offer updates on new standards, techniques, or technologies as well as issues the professional nurse is concerned with such as patient safety, error recovery, difficult communication, or working with diversity. Outside educational opportunities are usually advertised through the staff development office. Take advantage of the educational offerings. Each state board requires the nurse earn yearly continuing education units (CEUs) to maintain their license. Many internal and most external educational programs offer CEUs. Make sure you keep record of the programs you attend and the CEUs offered. With rapid changes in health care, it is critical for the nurse to keep abreast of the evidence that will provide the best patient care. A mentor can also provide the new nurse with teaching, coaching, and support.

FINDING A MENTOR

As each novice nurse eases into their new position, they have the opportunity to identify potential mentors. The difference between a preceptor and mentor is that a preceptor is assigned by a manager, whereas a mentor is a match that the new nurse identifies as someone who he/she feels comfortable learning from. Sometimes the preceptor turns out to be a mentor, but often the new nurse finds her own mentor by teaming up with different nurses. The mentor has a desire to share knowledge and time to offer support. The mentor carves out time of an already busy schedule to meet with the new nurse to establish a relationship where the goals of the new nurse are identified and a plan is designed to accomplish those goals. Eileen Hayes (2001) defined mentoring as "a voluntary committed, dynamic, extended, intense and supportive relationship characterized by trust, friendship and mutuality for the purpose of socializing students and promoting self efficacy" (p. 111). These are the mentor characteristics to look for:

1. Have a vested interest in the students success.
2. Love to teach.
3. Give students opportunities to learn by having confidence in their ability.
4. Offer humanistic feedback in a positive manner.
5. Share experiences, generate energy, and enthusiasm for the students future career.
6. Create the desire to continue a friendship.
7. Are life jackets that help protégés through difficult experiences.
8. Demonstrate they value beginning nurses through patience and kindness.
9. Provide role modeling.
10. Offer career advice.

In today's complex health care environment, mentors are seen as essential to the retention of the novice nurse. Many organizations have developed formal mentoring programs and some leave the mentoring process up to the individual. You can identify a mentor on your own by working with various nurses, asking the manager for suggestions, and checking with the departmental secretary for suggestions.

You also have something to offer the mentor. I have described the mutual benefit between mentor and protégé as collaborative mentoring, where both parties can learn from working with each other (Chandler, 2005). For example, recently a new nurse demonstrated to their mentor the efficacy of a PDA program. As a result, the mentor purchased their own PDA and was guided in its use by the new nurse.

Mentoring is a process that is learned and takes time to develop. Yet, in the busy world of nursing, senior nurses can adopt a mentoring attitude, recognizing that their life will be easier when new nurses join the team and are able to function to full capacity. There can be *mentoring moments* for each of us that can occur as you walk down the hall together. Pass the good news on.

EXPERIENCE AND ENVIRONMENT

Even with comprehensive orientations and expert preceptors, it is still a leap into practice and the recognition that it takes experience, experience one gains over time to move toward expertise. The novice nurse study (Ebright, Urdan, Patterson and Chalko, 2004) suggested the same recommendations from senior students listed in Chapter 5: organize, manage your time, and count on your friends. The good news is you have done this before, you have the skills from your experience as a student nurse, remember? Dee offers critical information to the new nurse on time management and focus:

I'm working on being more efficient with my time. I still forget to bring a saline flush and labels when I'm hanging IV antibiotics. The trip back to the med room takes another 3 minutes away from the time I could be doing something else. Those 3 minutes add up in the course of a shift. Neuro assessments take me a little while too. I had to refamiliarize myself with the 12 cranial nerves because the neurology residents want to know much more than is the patient A+O x 3, for example, is PERRLA intact, patient able to move all extremities, any right or left sided weakness, speech slur, facial drooping, can patient follow commands, do they have loss of appetite because they can't smell food?

I can think of many more times when I've felt incompetent and frustrated in my short month and half of working as a registered nurse but I don't think the stories themselves count. For me, what does count is focus. I say this to myself all the time. If you want to be a good nurse or be good at what you do, whatever it is, you have to be prepared to learn. Unfortunately, part of learning involves making mistakes. If you can accept that without wondering if, maybe you should have been a fashion designer, then you're on the right track.

Dee also reminds us, through all of your transition, do try to keep a sense of humor! Alena recognizes the gradual steps it takes to move into practice:

"If you don't hurt someone in the ICU you have done a good job." As my teacher said these words my heart stopped. At Oregon Health Sciences University (OHSU) my patients are so complex, so acute, and have survived some of the most intense surgeries. They are not exactly dying but rather trying to survive. The heart and its vasculature are so complex and for these patients are manipulated by an endless list of comorbidities. Sometimes I want to pull my patients' skin back to see first hand what we desperately seek in the monitors. I know it sounds grotesque but that way if someone asked me whether the patient was "wet" or "dry" I could say, "they are wet . . . see? and there is fluid in the lungs . . see? Let's give some Lasix." However, the body is not transparent. Once the body shows signs of distress it is at times at the last moment or even too late. It is up to the nurses to catch those crackles or temperature spikes because the symptoms might only last a moment before the body covers it up.

The body doesn't show symptoms the way you learned in nursing school. A person with a pulmonary embolism won't show signs of tachycardia if they are on beta blockers. A patient on sedation cannot say to the nurse, "I have an impending sense of doom." In the ICU, this body is manipulated by us and can't express itself in the ways that we have been taught. This is one of the scariest things about critical care. Yet, nurses learn. They learn through years of experiencing patient after patient. I may have the hard facts, the research, and the theory to save people but there is no substitute for a nurse's intuition and experience.

As a brand new nurse, Alena already recognizes what it takes to move from a novice to expert: experience, experience, experience plus a learning environment, where questions are welcomed and problem solving is collaborative. As Amanda progressed from orientation to being on her own, she realized the independence that comes with the new nurse role. The last time we heard from Amanda, she was worried that someone would end up dead when she was off orientation and on her own. Since then, she has learned how to assess the patient situation:

Luckily, I was wrong. Eleven weeks later, I have been off of orientation for one week. The most difficult thing I encountered was learning I would be making a lot of small decisions by myself. Little things that I would normally ask my nursing school instructor or preceptor at my internship like, "Should I give Tylenol? The patient's temp is 102?" Obviously! "Oh my god! The patient's blood pressure dropped! What do I do?" Assess, assess, assess!

I have learned that all those times in nursing school that I freaked out because I didn't have a chance to do some technical skill such as catheterizing or suctioning were completely unnecessary. Learning how to assess and critically think are all things that I learned and didn't realize I was learning it at the time. Now, as an official nurse taking care of her very own patients I am able to stop freaking out for a minute and think, "What could the problem be here?" and figure out what to do from there. Most importantly, I am never actually by myself. I am surrounded by other wonderful nurses and am given spectacular CNAs to work with. For every question I've ever had, there was always someone to turn to. Not a day goes by that I don't learn something new, and for that I am grateful because it will only make me a better nurse tomorrow.

The environment that you work in has a huge impact on your progress in nursing. Remember the things in the environment that empower the nurse: the right information, the appropriate amount of support, available resources, learning opportunities, and good relationships. Make sure that you have the resources you need to be empowered to practice. Amanda observed that her nursing ability was a product of her work environment, "I am surrounded by exceptional nurses and I am given spectacular CNAs to work with." Your nurse colleagues are the key to your success. Every nurse, new or seasoned, needs experienced nurses to consult with. Jodi, an RN out of school for 6 months, acknowledged, "The RNs I work with are really wonderful, many have been here for 30 years." Although there are many fine nurses, not everyone is an ideal colleague. You already know this from your student experience. Sue Roberts (1994) writes about nurses who feel like they have little power and influence in the medical hierarchy so turn their frustrations onto themselves and each other. Martha Griffin (2004) developed a program for new nurses to help them notice when the subtleties of relating to other nurses such as a caustic remark or a disapproving look became a barrier to the new nurse asking questions and learning from experienced staff. Griffin offers suggestions on how new nurses can protect themselves from these negative experiences by recognizing and confronting offensive behavior. But this sort of assertiveness takes practice. Many places offer classes in dealing with difficult situations.

See Dr. Griffin's article in the end of chapter reference list for more information on managing relationships with colleagues.

Paying attention to the environment in which you will work is an important aspect of taking a new job. During the job interview process, it is essential to notice the tone of the unit. This is difficult to do when you are so worried about how you are being judged, but the recruitment phase is your opportunity to make some judgments of your own. The larger system influences everything you will do on your new job. Whether the nurses work well together, whether the health care team truly collaborates, whether administration is talked in "us versus them" terms or if you are all working together to achieve the best possible patient care. Melissa is aware of the influence of the environment on her practice:

I think I've always been a "big picture" kind of person and every day I work on the floor I am always seeing things that could be different and if they were, could really improve the quality of patient care, patient & staff satisfaction, and the overall smoothness of running a big operation. I have done my best to keep my "voice," and have made it a point to introduce myself to key staff at the hospital that I talk to about my experiences as not only a new grad nurse but also a new person in the facility.

Developing and using your unique voice is the key to providing good patient care and essential to your success as a nurse. You bring a lot to the table even if it is simply questioning the accepted ways of work. You have about a year to preface every question you think is too bold or too dumb, by saying, "I know I am only new here but I was wondering . . ." and you can say anything! The questions from a nurse are critical to the care patients receive. Questioning is using the critical thinking you learned in school. The individual nursing voice and the collective voice of nurses is critical to patient care and system functioning. Recent reports have documented the importance of the nursing role in patient safety. The results of Aiken, Clarke, and Sloane's study (2002) indicate that the RN staffing level has significant effect on nurse surveillance. With an appropriate level of surveillance, the nurse is in the position to make direct assessments and initiate life-saving interventions, which can result in a decrease of preventable hospital deaths.

Ongoing professional development from orientation to grad rounds to formal education and certification programs can support the development of your knowledge your competence and confidence. Melissa, only after 6 months, already sees the need for more education to influence health care at the level that will make a difference:

Another thing I know you will be happy to hear is that the more I work on the floor, the more I want to go back to school and continue my education!

Stay tuned for the next chapter!

CONCLUSION

Moving into practice takes a village. You cannot make the transition on your own; you need a supportive environment, sensitive management, nurturing preceptors, potential mentors, and connections with peers. Nursing is not an individual practice. You need to be able to act on your own but depend on each other. That interdependence starts in your first nursing job.

END-OF-CHAPTER EXERCISE

Consider your future career from your first year after graduation to 5 to 10 years from now. When you develop a vision for your future, you will notice conversations and connections that will help you move toward that future. For example, you may be asked to be on a task force that will give you the opportunity to interact with experienced nurses from other floors. This could open up new horizons.

Try filling in the Career Goals table (Table 6-1) to anticipate the skills, connections, and education that you may need for the future.

Table 6-1. Career Goals

	First year	2–4 years	5–10 years	Additional skills, connections, and education
Possible career goals				
Personal goals				
Financial goals				
Future interests				

References

Aiken, L., Clarke, S., & Sloane, D. (2002). Hospital staffing, organization and quality of care: Cross national findings. *International Journal of Quality of Health Care*, *14*(1), 5–13.

Benner, P. (1984). *From novice to expert.* CA: Addison-Wesley Publishing Company.

Bridges, W. (1980). *Transitions.* Reading, MA: Addison-Wesley Publishing Company.

Chandler, G. (2005). Growing nurse leaders: An undergraduate teaching assistant program. *Journal of Nursing Education, 44*(12), 569–572.

Ebright, P., Urdan, L., Patterson, E., & Chalko, B. (2004). Themes surrounding novice nurse near-miss and adverse-event situation. *Journal of Nursing Administration, 34*(11), 531–538.

Firth, K., Sewell, J., & Clark, D. (2006). Best practices in NCLEX preparation for baccalaureate student success. *Nurse Educator,* May–June Supplement, 46S–53S.

Griffin, M. (2004). Teaching cognitive rehearsal as a shield for lateral violence: An intervention for newly licensed nurses. *Journal of Continuing Education in Nursing, 35*(6), 257–263.

Hayes, E. (2001). Factors that facilitate or hinder mentoring in the nursepractitioner preceptor/student relationship. *Clinical Excellence for NursePractitioners.* (5)2, 111–118.

Lauchner, K., Newman, M., & Britt, R. (2006). Predicting licensure success with a computerized comprehensive nursing exam: The HESI exit exam. *Nurse Educator,* May–June Supplement, 4S–9S.

Nibert, A., & Young, A. (2006). The third study on predicting NCLEX success with the HESI exit exam. *Nurse Educator,* May–June Supplement, 21S–27S.

Nibert, A., Young, A., & Adamson, C. (2006). Predicting NCLEX success with the HESI exit exam: Fourth annual validation study. *Nurse Educator,* May–June Supplement, 28S–34S.

Roberts, S. (1994). Oppressed group behaviors: Implications for nursing. *Revolution,* Fall, 29–35.

Tucker, A., & Edmundson, A. (2002). Managing routine exceptions: A model of nurse problem solving behavior. *Advances in Health Care Management, 3,* 87–113.

CHAPTER 7

Going Back

Anticipating Graduate School

Some students know before they even graduate from their baccalaureate program that they will be going back for their Master's degree. They recognize that the undergraduate program prepared them to be a nurse generalist and one of their career goals is to specialize in an area of nursing they have already set their sights on. That was not me. As I was graduating from my 4-year program, at the age of 21, I swore I would never go back to school.

It was a bright sunny day in Buffalo, New York. This was weather I had not seen in this western New York city since I had never stuck around until late May during my 4 years of incarceration. But this year was different. After eight semesters of intense studying, early morning clinicals, and late night partying, I was ready to receive my baccalaureate diploma. Alleluia! I never thought this day would come.

Donning our caps and gowns we lined up for our practice procession in Klinehans' Music Hall. In alphabetical order our all female class filed into the rows of deep maroon cushioned seats. As we waited for our next instructions one of our faculty asked us, "Who is going on to graduate school?" There were a few whispers, "Oh yeah, right!" Without even looking up we all knew which of our peers would raise their hands. The same girls that volunteered to help the nuns on weekends, the usual goody two shoes that ran for student government (my position as class senator being the exception), those half a dozen students who always jumped when faculty called would raise their hands to go to graduate school. Shaking our heads at the ridiculousness of the question, I declared, "I am never, ever going back to school!"

Two years later, after being a staff nurse and eyeing the head nurse position, I was filling out a graduate school application for a clinical nurse specialist program. After moving into management, less than 18 months after I received my graduate degree, I was heading for a certificate program for Nurses in Management at Harvard School of Public Health. Watching the psychology graduate students getting funded to conduct research on the unit, I decided I needed a PhD four years after the certificate. I was the first PhD of my undergraduate class! Never say never.

So those few of my peers that raised their hands back in the music hall may have known something I didn't. Then again, I was just not ready to commit to more school. When the time is right, graduate school is a good idea. You might want to consider it.

WHAT'S IN IT FOR YOU?

Good question. Why go back to school when you can make a good salary where you are and you already feel pretty confident about your knowledge and skills? Confidence and competence is what many nurses feel in practice but some still wonder what else is out there? Susan talks about her experience as a young BS graduate:

I was 21 years old, in my first year working as a nurse on a consulting medical floor in a large teaching hospital. Our patients were cared for by a variety of attending physicians—cardiologists, pulmonologists, nephrologists, neurologists, and gastroenterologists. I was so focused on the clinical issues I needed to learn that it took me a while to figure out who the players were around me. One day I noticed a woman rounding with the cardiology attending and fellows. We had a conversation about a patient, and I asked who she was. "I'm a clinical nurse specialist in cardiology," she said. I hadn't heard about nurse specialists, but I was intrigued. I asked questions, and I watched her for months after that. What I saw was intelligence and quiet respect for her as a part of the cardiology team. The image of the clinical nurse specialist stayed with me for three more years as I worked on other units in the hospital, always feeling vaguely dissatisfied with where I was and what I was doing. When I was ready to go to graduate school, I knew that what I was looking for could be found in the role of nurse specialist or nurse practitioner.

Susan was looking toward her future, contemplating a career that would grow and change with her. There are several areas of concentration for nurse practitioners including adult acute care, adult health, family, pediatric, oncology, neonatal, gerontology, and women's health, to name a few. A list of accredited graduate schools can be found at http://www.nursingsociety.org/education/schoolsUS.html.

Bill considered graduate school after the RN Mobility program, when he wondered what else was there inside of him that he is not challenging yet:

My journey through the RN to BS program was much more than I anticipated. Initially, I believed I would read, complete assignments, progress from course to course and graduate. While that did occur, I never anticipated the impact of the effects my relationship with faculty would have on me. I was encouraged, supported, motivated, and challenged. In return, I gained confidence and strong desire to do more and go further with my education.

Note that the encouragement and support came through in an **RN Mobility** all online program. Although many contemplate taking that first step to graduate school by earning a Bachelor's degree through an online format, the efficacy and the connection of online learning is still questioned. As an online convert, who said it couldn't be done, my recommendation is, as with any program, you need to do your research. I believe, just as Bill did, you'll find an online program that will work for you.

For those students with a **baccalaureate degree in another field,** there are many options that can lead to a graduate degree. There are second-entry programs that allow you to earn a Bachelor's degree in nursing in a year to 18 months with the same amount of clinical hours as a traditional undergraduate program (see Chapters 2 and 3). Then there are several **fast track programs** for the student with a baccalaureate outside of nursing to go straight through graduate school. The undergraduate studies typically take a year with the addition of a year and a half in a graduate specialty program. According to American Association of Colleges of Nursing ([AACN] 2006), currently there are programs in 43 states with 173 second degree programs and 46 Master's programs.

GRADUATE SCHOOL

The official goal of graduate education, according to the AACN Essential of Masters Education (1996) document, is to develop "the ability to critically and accurately assess, plan, intervene, and evaluate health and illness experiences of clients (individuals, families and communities)." In schools accredited by AACN there must be a Graduate Core Curriculum and Advanced Practice Core Curriculum.

The Graduate Core Curriculum content includes:

1. Research
2. Health Organization, Policy, and Finance
3. Ethics
4. Role Development
5. Theoretical Foundations of Nursing Practice
6. Human Diversity and Social Issues
7. Health Promotion and Disease Prevention

The Advanced Practice Core Curriculum content includes:

1. Advanced Health and Physical Assessment
2. Advanced Physiology and Pathophysiology
3. Advanced Pharmacology

Okay, so that looks like a lot. Some may interest you, some may not. Don't be deterred. There are several approaches to learning more about what you might like to study:

- To build your enthusiasm about learning more in your specialty, go directly to the literature, head for the library, or go to the electronic database of CINAHL or PubMed, and look into what is being talked about in your area of interest.
- If you have not already, consider joining a specialty organization to keep up on what is new; http://www.nursingsociety.org/career has a list of all the specialty sites.
- Attend a nursing conference. Learn about what is current and what the future is in your area of interest. Conferences are mind expanding and great fun! You meet a lot of interesting people and have the opportunity to build professional networks. You will definitely get a feel for what focus in your specialty you'd like to learn more about *and* meet the people who are studying in that area. Researchers are always interested in talking to people who are interested in their

research. The material presented at conferences is peer reviewed, meaning a panel of peers decided whether the presentation was based on solid evidence, good research, and is current. Hearing about cutting-edge material can help you decide whether you are ready to pursue further education.

The decision to return to school is a life-changing choice. Nurses recognize the need for graduate education at different points in their career. Today there are many fast track options that take you right from your undergraduate degree to a PhD, the research degree, or the DNP, the Doctorate of Nursing Practice. Early in my career I realized that I needed a graduate degree despite my pompous proclamations after my undergrad program:

I was working in my dream job in one of the top three psychiatric facilities in the country. I had started in psych, went to med-surg and primarily due to my interest in being treated as an equal member of the health care team, I came back to psych. Here, the nurse worked with patients, met with families, and managed medications 24/7. The nurse was viewed not only as an equal but looked up to for the knowledge and experience with patient care. However, day after day of sitting in clinical conferences and reviewing treatment plans with my esteemed colleagues I recognized that everyone around the table had specialty training but me. The social worker had a graduate degree, the psychologist had a doctoral degree and the physician had a medical degree with a specialty in psychiatry. Now I'll admit, I am a quick study, but I wanted to know more about psychiatric-mental health nursing so I could fully bring the nursing perspective to the discussion. I needed a specialty degree in nursing. Back to school.

Graduate degrees are offered in different specialty areas for a Clinical Nurse Specialist (CNS), a Clinical Nurse Leader (CNL), or a Nurse Practitioner (NP). A full-time clinical nurse specialist program is usually 2 years long, and you specialize in a particular area of nursing with the goal of working in an acute or long-term care facility. There are many different roles for a CNS from working on a specialty unit consulting to the staff nurses to working through the education department to consulting throughout the facility. The psych/mental health CNS program met my immediate career goals because I wanted to continue to work on an inpatient unit and provide consultation throughout the hospital. The CNL degree fit Bill's aspirations. With a strong practice background as a 2-year AD nurse, Bill came right into graduate school after the RN Mobility program. He chose the CNL program:

As I reviewed the graduate programs I was intrigued by the courses titled, "advanced." This was another milestone. I asked myself, "Do I have what it takes to succeed in a graduate class?" With some trepidation, I enrolled. And, so far, I have succeeded. Again, the result of incredible guidance and support from faculty.

For some students, obtaining an advanced degree is necessary for their pursuit of advanced practice. For me, my desire for obtaining an advanced degree is for more education. My goal was initially obtaining a BS in nursing. As a result of the effects that the nursing faculty had on me, I was not only challenged to continue with my education, I was given the encouragement and support that enabled me to take a risk and succeed in graduate school.

Bill did the research necessary to locate the program and the faculty that fit his educational needs and career aspirations. The CNL concentration prepares nurses to design, provide, and manage health promotion, risk reduction, and illness management for individuals and clinical populations. The CNL works across clinical settings, collaborates with other disciplines, and coordinates patient care. Some nurses return to school for reasons close to the heart. Rozy chose to study for a Family Nurse Practitioner degree for the pursuit of knowledge and to honor her heritage:

I am Mexican-American. I grew up very poor. Many doors were closed to me. We had few possessions, and, at times, we had no food. But there was a local library where I could check out books for free. I would check out ten books, the maximum, every week. I loved the books about young women who would defy the odds living in poverty and go on to scale mountains in education. My father never went to school. My mother went as far as the 8th grade. They were so proud of me for doing well in school. I am the first one in my family with a four year degree. I also wanted to get my Master's to honor my parents, and, in some way, to honor my heritage. I can open so many more doors now.

Rozy was one of my Teaching Assistants. I can attest to her success in graduate studies and anything else she sets her mind to.

There are also advanced practice programs in Nurse-Midwifery, Nurse Anesthetist, Administration, and in Education. There are several dual degree options combining an MS in nursing with a Master's in public health or a Master's in business. After analyzing the graduate school options in mid-career, There is a choice to return to school for a Master's in nursing education:

Graduate school? I must be crazy! At almost 50 years old, why would I commit myself (and my family) to the financial obligation, the study time or the computer practice I will need to bone up on to pull this off? (The final paper for my last degree program was a type written *paper!) A thousand reasons why, but one primary driving force behind my decision, is the satisfaction I get from sharing my love of nursing with others.*

In 2003, I was given the opportunity to teach a clinical practicum group for a nursing program. After two and half years of teaching new nursing students I could envision myself doing this more often than on a casual basis.

I found motivation from family, nursing peers, students, and the education program director. I mapped out a time line (did I mention I am a type A personality who likes to have all of her ducks in a row?) and looked at budgeting and potential programs. I attended an informational open house which was presented by area colleges. I spoke with recruiters and collected a litany of material in the form of booklets and pamphlets, which outlined coursework and prerequisites. I spoke with respected educators regarding graduate programs they had attended and asked them what the deciding factors were in selecting their nursing paths. I found I had at least one thing in common with them, a fundamental love of nursing and the need to share my knowledge and skills with others seeking the same rewards.

I selected one of the programs which provided me the option of taking 5 years to complete the degree requirements (remember my time line?). I selected a program which specifically offered a Master's in nursing education. Aha, just the focus for what I was intent on practicing.

Theresa did her research and found a graduate program that met her current career aspirations. Doing the research to find a program that fits is one of the initial steps to an advanced degree.

FIRST STEP

We know that to feel empowered one needs the right information, the right resources, the right support, and the right relationships (Chandler, 1991). Looking into to graduate school begins with taking time to listen to that internal voice and identify your future goals. You will need to decide what

your passion is in nursing: is it teaching? Becoming an expert in a specialty area? Or developing an autonomous nursing practice in primary care?
The first step to advanced education is finding your passion.

The Right Information

The first information you need comes from within, discovering what your
passion in nursing is. A passion is critical considering that at times graduate school can be difficult, frustrating, and tedious. You must have that
passion that will create the drive to work through the challenges and press
forward to reach your goal. Bill's attention to his voice steered him back to
graduate school:

*When I first began completing the requirements for the RN to BS program I
viewed my graduation as the culmination to a long sought after goal. I must
acknowledge that I was surprised by my thoughts and emotions as graduation
came closer. Something within me, perhaps my internal voice, was suggesting that
this in fact was not the end of the journey towards my goal; rather, a continuation
of a journey steeped in education, self-exploration, trust, and risk taking.*

Some nurses are so passionate about their practice that they feel like they
need to know more to provide the best patient care. Rozy talks about her
internal drive:

*One of my favorite challenges in nursing is the need to know more. We need to
know more about new medications, procedures, the disease process, and
research: the medical sky is the limit! I believe knowledge is power, and I
wanted the knowledge and the power to decide more for my patients. I knew
I could do this by becoming a nurse practitioner, an advanced practice nurse.
I never liked saying, "I don't know" when asked a question by a patient, a
family member, or another health care worker. Of course, I cannot know
"everything," but again, I wanted to know more. I wanted to hear from and
to learn from other nurses who had furthered their education. It seems like
such a gift, this sharing of knowledge and experience. I wanted, but knew I
could not have, ALL the experiences these nurses in graduate school had. But
I could sure learn from their experience.*

Holle talks about having accumulated a wealth of experience in clinical
practice over the last 8 years and was now wondering, what next?

I made the decision to go back to school after I'd been working on the oncology unit for about 7 or 8 years. I'd reached that "what am I going to do with the rest of my career/life?" question. I felt I'd mastered the floor nurse/oncology thing and found myself bored at work. I continued to read and stay current in my specialty and was frustrated when other nurses around me seemed to be going through the motions, not willing to learn or explore new ideas. Could I continue the 12-hour shifts as I got older, was there room for growth?

Other nurses hear of an opportunity to be funded to further their knowledge and skills. For example, there may be a new gerontology program starting up at the university that is funded by a grant that includes tuition and a stipend. Or a program may be government-funded if you contract to provide health care in an underserved area for 2 years after graduation. The opportunity to have your education funded may come at a time in your career that you could consider graduate school. Eileen started out as an LPN:

I have "taken the scenic route" through my nursing education. A lot of what happened over the course of my education happened because I am a female, a life partner, and a mother. In many ways, nursing is a quintessential woman's profession, and because of that, there are many opportunities to pursue education and work circumstances that will fit around the hundred-and-one other roles that women take on. I parsed out my education and my nursing career to fit around my life as a wife and mother. Of course, this is exactly what keeps most women and nurses at the lower end of the earning and achievement totem-pole, but that's a different story.

I actually started out as a pre-med student—my first 2 years at B.U. had that as the ultimate goal. At the time, B.U. had an experimental (and short-lived) 6-year med program—I thought that's what I wanted. Then I found out I could do as nurse what I thought I wanted to do as a physician. Nursing had that added appeal of a fundamentally different way of looking at people and life and health that resonated with me. Then I got married and had a couple of babies, moved around the country as a Navy wife, and didn't get back to my education for another 5 years. I started as an LPN, because at the time (we were stationed in Connecticut at the Sub Base in Groton) there was a nursing shortage and the State of Connecticut paid for me to go to school. I got my Associate degree at HCC when they introduced a streamlined LPN to ADN track. From there I attended the RN to BS program.

My entry into the Master's track was influenced by a couple of circumstances. The first is my interest in pursuing advanced preparation in nursing, for my own practice and so that I will also be able to teach at some point. My travels through academia and different nursing settings made me realize how important it is to mentor new nurses, and to teach them how to practice mindfully. So many nurses don't practice this way, and far too many practice sites don't encourage or value mindful practice. I want to do my part to change that. The other circumstance that precipitated my return to the Master's program was the availability of grant monies to fund the educational aspirations of new nursing faculty. Conversations with a senior faculty member brought me back into the fold. I have to say that without that funding, I couldn't and likely wouldn't have been able to return.

The value of nursing, faculty mentoring, nurse-to-nurse mentoring, and developing a mindful practice are all good reasons to return to graduate school. Learn more information about programs through school informational sessions. Most schools offer informational sessions that can be very helpful for learning about specific program requirements, meeting the school representatives, connecting to other interested applicants, and the opportunity to meet current students in the program and alumni who have graduated recently. Frequently, informational sessions are offered in health care facilities, so ask your education office for updates on school programs. For the potential applicant or the vaguely intrigued visitor, an informational session can provide you with food for thought and expand your network of connections. Check out the school web sites for times and locations of informational meetings. Before attending the session, thoroughly review the program's web site so that you can come prepared with questions to make the best use of the time. The fact that we have a desperate faculty shortage also may provide individual impetus and government funding to support returning to school, so make sure to ask about funding for school.

The Right Resources

Once you have a notion of what your interest is, then you can get practical with where you want to go to school, how much it'll cost, and how long will it take. School web sites will answer many of the questions you have and an actual in-person information session should take care of the rest of your concerns. You have to ask yourself whether you can move across the country or are you geographically bound? There are graduate schools in the inner city, in the desert, in private colleges, and at most state universities.

Graduate school is a great time to explore working with unique populations in different parts of the country.

After a quick scan of graduate program possibilities, begin to calculate the resources you will need to support your decision to return to school. Here are some questions to guide you in considering resources:

- Are there grants connected to the program you are interested in?
- Does the school have teaching assistantships (TA) and research assistantships (RA) for graduate students that fund graduate student tuition?
- Will a TA be guaranteed for your entire program or just the first year?
- Does your current place of employment provide for tuition reimbursement?
- Are there stipends that the school gives to your organization that you can apply for? For instance, some schools give tuition waivers for being able to use the site for undergraduate clinical experiences. The individual nurse just needs to apply for the waiver.
- What scholarships do nursing specialty organizations offer?

In addition to capital resources, you will need family, friends, and work support to start down the educational path.

The Right Support

Your family can be a huge source of support, or not, so make sure that they know about your desire to return to school. Your family needs to be on board so that each individual can anticipate their role in support of your decision. Your partner's role will most likely expand to fill in for your responsibilities, your kids will have to pitch in, your relatives may be called on. Remember Monica and Susan in Chapter 5 talked about sharing their research and writing with their college age children? The new roles can be growth producing for all!

Connecting to your network of personal and professional friends that you identified in Chapter 6 will be helpful in sorting through options and listening to your rationale for going back to school. Active membership in one of the 100 nurse specialty organizations can provide a network of individuals to consult with on your career interests (http://www.nursingsociety. org/career).

Once you have identified your specialty area of interest and the schools in your range of possibilities, go to the school's web site to learn about the mission, vision, and values of programs you are interested in. In graduate school, you will work more closely with individual faculty, so it is important to read about faculty interests and accomplishments on the web site. Pay particular attention to the descriptions of practice interventions and research programs that get you excited: a focus on AIDS research? A program on Alternative Medicine? A Center for Women's Health? A program in Rehabilitation nursing? How do these specific programs fit with your career goals?

Now we are getting closer to actually visiting a campus. A friend who recently entered a grad program said he wished he had visited the schools earlier in his decision making. Reflecting back, he observed that from the interaction with faulty and the feel of the campus he would have known immediately that certain programs would not have made his preferred list. Before you show up in person, though, consider the following warning: be aware that visiting a campus or even reading graduate school web sites may incur the commonly felt feelings of the imposter syndrome.

The Imposter Syndrome

The human side of considering graduate school is the hidden concern about whether you are good enough to be accepted into a graduate program. Let's face it, when many nurses think about returning for their Bachelor's, Master's, or doctoral degree, they hear that gnawing internal critic asking the question, "Am I smart enough to handle graduate school?" The answer is worth considering. "Smart" is a word used to describe many assets, from IQ to emotional intelligence to your aspirations and drive.

 Reflection 1: Are You Smart Enough?

That is:

1. How did the prerequisite courses go?

2. Have you studied enough for the GREs?

3. Are you ready to take on the work that will change your lifestyle? Your worldview? Your professional and personal relationships?

4. Do you have the motivation, persistence, and support to make the commitment to graduate school?

These are important pragmatic questions to consider. Some you can take care of right away by signing up for a GRE in-person or online/review course. Or, if you are disciplined enough, get the GRE study book and develop a daily study plan. Then there are the middle of the night questions that pop up: *will they be able to tell I am not smart enough?* You recognize who I am talking about: That critic that peeks its head out as you lay your head down on the pillow, or that internal voice that is so deeply ingrained it has the power to wake you up in the middle of the night from a sound sleep, or that fraudulent feeling that hovers over you as you lay staring at the ceiling in the gray light just before dawn. Everyone has an internal critic whose full-time job is to hold you back. Anne Lamott (1995), a very successful author, talks about her experience of the internal critic that rises up just as she sits down to write:

Your mental illnesses arrive at the desk like your sickest, most secretive relative. And they pull up chairs in a semi-circle around your computer, and they try to be quiet but you know they are there with their weird coppery breath, leering at you behind your back . . . . First I try to breathe, because I am either sitting there panting like a lap dog or I am unintentionally making slow asthmatic death rattles. So I just sit there a minute, breathing slowly, quietly. I let my mind wander. After a moment I may notice that I am trying to decide whether I am too old for orthodontia and whether right now would be a good time to make a few calls, and then I start to think about learning how to use makeup . . .

All of this happens just as she is about to start the first page of her new novel. You get the picture. We've all been there. The internal critic throws up barriers, begs for procrastination, and can let you know at every turn that you are not smart enough for this next move. We allow the internal critic in when we are feeling like we might not belong in graduate school. This critic is most likely a symptom of the imposter syndrome. The syndrome that makes one feels like they don't belong, they are not good enough, they are fakes or frauds. The results of the syndrome can paralyze individuals from moving forward or at least have them apologize for not being smart enough or deserving enough to be in the positions they aspire to. "This probably isn't right but I was thinking . . ." "This doesn't sound very good but I'll read it anyways . . . " You may not agree with me, but . . . " These common statements represent fraudulent feelings that come from feeling like you are in the wrong place, somehow you have snuck in, you may be found out, someone will report the C you got in high school biology. Peg McIntosh (1985) wrote a paper entitled "Feeling Like A Fraud" that discusses the dynamics that enable the imposter syndrome. McIntosh writes, "I suggest that on the one hand feeling like a fraud indicates that we have, deplorably, internalized value systems that said most people were incompetent and illegitimate in the spheres of power and public life and authority. But, then on the other hand, I suggest that when we apologize in public, we are at some level making a deeply wise refusal to carry on the pretense of deserving and feeling good about roles in conventional and oppressive hierarchies." She recommends that fraudulence should be analyzed politically and suggests that feeling like a fraud should be applauded because it sets the stage for social action and political change.

So let's consider this advice. You are trying to find the time and energy to apply to an institution of higher education but other things come up, like your son's dental appointment or your aunt's sudden illness or learning how to use makeup, anything that can keep you from seriously even considering the application. Okay, now we know that is our internal critic and we need to put it to rest so we can get serious about grad school. Then there is the feeling like you don't belong there anyway. We will not measure up. We will not fit in. As one who has spent the majority of my career in the university setting I'd have to agree with McIntosh, there are rigid hierarchies that are difficult to access. There are inner circles that do not have many people that look like me. There is little room at the top. This situation should not stop you from moving on but, rather, have you question what it is that is so special or separate about the inner circle. We certainly all know at the highest forms of government, which are very exclusive and filled with so-called smart people, there is blatant corruption and planned deceit. I also agree that the personal feelings of fraudulence have meaning at some level: "We are making a deeply wise refusal to carry on the pretense of deserving and feeling good about roles in conventional and oppressive hierarchies." Our sense of not belonging and of being kept out may be telling us something about the agenda of the inner sanctum. These hierarchies are select and disempowering. Once you acknowledge the feelings of the imposter syndrome may serve a purpose, listen to this voice, use the feelings to your benefit, but do not let them stop you from moving forward. In every returning RN, second Bachelor's, Master's, and doctoral class that I have taught, the individual students sitting around the table who have rearranged work schedules and delegated family obligations, drove many miles and found a parking place or those online students sitting alone at a remote site at their computer, began with feeling out of their element until they recognized everyone in the room had similar feelings. In fact, these fellow graduate students sitting around the real or virtual table have very similar career aspirations to you. They have felt different from their work colleagues for awhile. They are not satisfied with the status quo and want more knowledge, advanced skills, and a broader perspective of the health care environment. They are juggling work and family and are more than likely members of the sandwich generation taking care of growing children and aging parents. These are your new peers. Listen to that imposter voice for what it is telling you and then move on to your next step in education. You have come to the right place!

WHAT IS GRADUATE SCHOOL LIKE?

Graduate school is exciting! Think about it. As an undergraduate, you worked hard to develop your skills as a generalist. Now, in graduate school, you will be studying in an area that *you* have chosen and area of nursing that *you* are passionate about. You will have the opportunity to conduct research on topics you've been curious about in your practice. You will have the opportunity to work with nurse experts, nurse scientists, and nursing leaders. Holle talks about her impression of graduate school:

Grad school was daunting, I knew I could do it, but did I need the extra pressure, the juggling of family and obligations? Roadblocks aside, I started, sweaty palms, upset stomach, the whole 9 yards, but I loved school, I loved the new knowledge base and challenging myself. My family was supportive, my friends didn't understand, some colleagues called me "ambitious" in snide asides, others told me I was taking on too much and probably grew tired of my constant turn downs of invitations . . . . I completed 2 years and then I had another crisis, did

I really want to leave the comfort and security of being a nurse to take on the overwhelming responsibilities of becoming an NP? Stay tuned.

It is exciting to anticipate reading, writing, and conducting research in the specialty area that fits your interest. That is a large part of graduate school. You will be assigned an extraordinary amount of reading to prepare for the time spent in class with a professor and your peers. Classes are generally 1 or 2 days/week to accommodate the family/working professional. Programs start with core courses in theory, research, and ethics/policy/current issues in nursing that every student takes. During the second year, students branch off into specialty areas with the support theory and clinical courses. Classes are much smaller and more interactive than undergraduate classes. There may be 10 to 20 students in a core course with fewer in the specialty classes. Many classes are in the form of seminars where students and faculty discuss the readings. You will be closer to your peers and your professors. Your professors and clinical preceptors will become advisors, mentors, and future colleagues. Holly, a PhD student, tells us about her initiation into graduate school:

I wondered how I would form relationships with my colleagues, my classmates. The first day of class was September 11, 2001 at 9 A.M. Our first class took place in a multimedia classroom so we would get used to the technology we would experience during the course of the year. Even before we took our seats, we were aware that a plane had hit one of the Twin Towers. This announcement was soon followed by the news of the other plane; at that point we began to attend to the TV, rather than the class. Here I was surrounded by strangers (we had met twice before), about 2 hours from home, unable to contact my family, and trying to figure out how and where to get books (I needed to go to three different places to get what I needed for class) to begin this journey. The next week started with us describing how we had felt about the events of the previous week. My comment, that this event would define us as a class, was met with agreement from all.

To be prepared for your scholarly discussions, there will be multiple assigned readings from nursing and related disciplines with the expectation that you will become familiar with the most recent evidence in the discipline and your specialty. While you are in school, you will learn about research evidence that will serve as a base for your future as an advanced practitioner. The skills you develop in reviewing the literature and understanding research studies are skills you will use every day in your nursing practice. The strategies for learning, such as reading, writing, presenting, research, and grant writing will serve you well. The new learning is both challenging and humbling. More than likely, you were an expert in practice and now you are about to become a student again, a student who has a lot to learn. The transition from expert to novice is an interesting journey and one where you can expect to go thorough the stages of socialization once again. First honeymoon and then the shock at the amount of work required, remember? You have been here before.

The reading in graduate school is plentiful and often overwhelming. The goal is to become an expert in the discipline, which requires a breadth and depth of reading. Several books and many articles will be assigned per course. When you first start back, it can feel like the required reading is in a foreign language. The concepts and style of presentation is very different from that of clinical practice. You will use the critical thinking you have developed in practice but applied to thinking critically about theories put forth by nurse experts and research conducted by nurse scientists. Holly's observation of being a new PhD student is often reiterated by all levels of graduate students:

There were volumes to read each week. Fortunately, I am a quick reader. However, some of the material was so obtuse that reading it was not necessarily helpful. I remember speaking to a former student of mine, who had returned to school to become a nurse as an adult. I asked her, "How are you standing feeling so stupid?" That is how I felt—stupid. There were so many things I knew nothing about. Here was what Benner spoke about in Novice to Expert. *I was no longer an expert, I was a novice.*

You will be expected to be able to express your own ideas and cite the evidence of experts in both oral and written communication. Active participation in face-to-face discussions and, in some classes, through virtual discussions, will be expected. In-class interactions will be built on your previous experience and your current reading. Out-of-class papers and projects are designed to increase your knowledge through becoming familiar with the literature. Citing scholar's ideas, comprehending a body of knowledge, and synthesizing your own thoughts into succinct, clear, academically written, and oral presentations are all skills that you will develop in grad school. My advice: start now. I mean go to the local college library and read the literature, visit the National Institutes of Health (NIH) site (http://www.nih.gov), visit the Center for Disease Control (CDC) site (http://www.cdc.gov), visit the Agency for Healthcare Research and Quality (AHRQ) site (http://www.ahrq.gov), and dust off your American

Psychological Association manual (APA) so that you can be ready to put it to use again (there is probably a new version and there are now actually many web sites that have what you will need to properly use APA format for writing papers). Writing papers in graduate school is a whole new level of thinking. The four goals of academic writing are:

1. To be able to locate appropriate evidence
2. To develop command of the subject
3. To develop the specialized literacy of academic writing
4. To develop cohesive texts

Most schools assume students will have reached the goal upon entry into the program. Yet, formal writing is a learned discipline that depends on understanding the theory and research language of the discipline. Thus, the extensive reading requirements to initiate students into encoded language of the nursing research community. Papers presented at professional meetings or published in professional journals are how researchers communicate to others in their field. Through coursework in methods and theory and interaction with faculty and peers, students are initiated into the research community. To learn how to communicate through the disciplines, written conventions students will have to progress from facts, "knowing that" to the application of the facts to a task, "knowing how" (Berkenkotter, Huckin, & Ackerman, 1988). This is no small task.

In graduate school, you should have ample time to practice the new skills you are learning in clinical placements under the guidance of faculty and the supervision of preceptors. Some schools provide placements; others encourage students to organize their own clinical experience. Some schools have local clinical experiences, whereas others offer international opportunities. Research each program carefully. Reread Chapter 4 on applications, essays and interviews. Your graduate application process should be more of a collaborative experience with the school where you take the initiative to find the program, the faculty, and the pedagogical style that meets your particular needs. The faculty will be interviewing you to decide how well you fit what the program has to offer and you will be interviewing the faculty to see if they fit your interests and goals (see Chapter 4). The graduate faculty will be your mentors. You are looking for a fit. What type of mentors have you had so far? From my research on empowerment (Chandler, 1991), I know that there are five essential components that are needed to experience empowerment: the right information, hands-on and emotional support, tangible resources, opportunities to test your abilities, and relationships that provide mentoring. Go down the list and make sure that you have what you need to be empowered to succeed in graduate school.

Reflection 2: Mentor Map

To learn more about what you are looking for in a graduate program, consider what has worked in the past:

• Who has advised you, coached you, and assisted you in growing in your career?

• Who could you go to for the information you needed?

• Who supports you personally in your career development? Who are your cheerleaders?

• Who can provide you with resources to do your job well?

• Who provides you with opportunities to try your wings and is there someone to support your flight?

• Who are your mentors? Who have you mentored?

Reflecting on your responses, what do you need both professionally and personally to be empowered to be successful in graduate school?

It is so important to take this opportunity to learn about what works for you so you can take the initiative to build on what you already know and create new networks where they are needed. It is useful to take stock of the support that you will need to succeed. One time when I was working on a writing intervention in a teen shelter, the writing prompt was to list what provides you with comfort and support in your life. The goal of the writing intervention was to facilitate self efficacy and self esteem (Chandler, 1999). I wrote with the adolescents and we all read our writing aloud while the others listened closely and commented on what they liked and what they remembered about the writing. We were using the Amherst Writers and Artists' method developed by Pat Schneider (2003). That night, sitting around the table in the shelter's well-worn kitchen, everyone wrote their story about comforts and supports. When I read what I wrote, the group members observed that although I was much less vulnerable than they were, I had the longest list of supports. Their comments were, "You do *that* many things for support?" I told them to juggle this life of family, work, and friends; it takes a cast of thousands, from child care, to friends, to book groups, to mentors, to therapists, to exercise. Shaking their heads in disbelief, they each vowed to expand on their own networks of support.

Reflection 3: What Does Your Network Look Like?

What or who do you need to build your network of:

- Information?

- Support?

- Resources?

- Opportunities?

- Relationships?

DOCTORAL PROGRAMS

Doctoral programs are either research-intensive, the PhD, or clinically focused, the Doctorate of Nursing Practice (DNP). The common theme in doctoral programs is that they prepare:

- Leaders
- Researchers
- Educators
- Clinical experts
- Public policy analysts

Doctorally prepared nurses work in executive positions, on university faculty, as health policy analysts, as researchers in health care institutions, and for government agencies.

The PhD

The PhD is a research degree with a focus on advancing nursing knowledge to improve practice, design, and use evidence-based data to address individual-, group-, and population-based health problems and to develop future educators and leaders. Similar to the Master's program, the PhD curriculum consists of core courses in research methods, theory, and state of the discipline followed by specialty courses in your area of interest. The focus of a given PhD program reflects the faculty's area of research. This means that you decide on a PhD program by the program focus and the faculty's research area. So first you identify a research area you would like to pursue and then you locate a faculty member who is conducting research in the area you are interested in. Your PhD program will consist of general courses, specialty courses, and working with a faculty mentor on your dissertation. You will want your mentor to be an expert in the area you want to study so that you can receive the guidance you need to begin a program of research. As a potential student, you want to find a match between your interests and the program's foci and a faculty's research area.

Just as with a Master's degree, students choose to come back to school for different reasons at different times of their life. Holly recalls:

I remember feeling I needed to wait until my daughters were "old enough" to return to school to get my PhD. Old enough to understand what I was doing, old enough to see me doing my own school work (not my home work as faculty). I was so excited about having this opportunity. I was so looking forward to the exchange of ideas between faculty and students. When I went to the UMass to find out about the program and when I returned for my interview I loved the dialogue. I thought, "This was going to be great!"

I, by contrast, decided on doctoral studies before I had children. Well, almost . . . :

I wanted to learn about the research process, learn how to obtain funding to support nursing research and teach at a university. The PhD would give me the knowledge and skills to pursue my goals. I started my PhD program in September and my first baby was born on November 12. Two years later, my daughter was born and 3 years after that, the same month I was defending my dissertation, I had my third child. As I like to say, I was the most productive student in the doctoral program!

The PhD program is intense, exhilarating, and paradigm-shifting. You will be challenged by your professors, your coursework, and your peers. Your thinking will move to another level. Your worldview will change. Holly admits:

While I found the qualitative research class challenging, I enjoyed reading the texts as well as the studies. But it was the philosophy of science class that was a real bear. It was not just about learning about content, it was learning about myself, my thoughts, values, and beliefs. My own philosophical under-pinnings were closely examined. And at times that could be somewhat painful. And when I tried to share what I had learned back at work with my nursing faculty colleagues, they were not interested in engaging in a discussion with me. Actually, it was the president of the college I worked for at the time with whom I had the most interesting dialogues.

While some of my classmates were pretty sensitive about receiving critique from the faculty, I welcomed it. I called it, "being on the other side of the red pen." I think that it helped me be a better teacher.

Not only will you be a better teacher but you will collaborate with faculty, conduct research, present at conferences, and publish the results. Watch out world, here I come!

The DNP offers a practice option.

The DNP

The Doctorate in Nursing Practice program is a response to the public's growing concern about health care quality, access, and disparities. The DNP provides the advanced knowledge and skills for the nurse clinician to address the increased complexity of health care, the focus on patient safety, and importance of patient outcomes. The DNP prepares nurses to practice at the highest level. Typically, DNP programs have coursework in advanced clinical knowledge, advanced skills, research translation, and leadership. With successful completion of the DNP program, the nurse is expected to use scientific knowledge from nursing and related disciplines to improve health outcomes, to collaborate with other health care leaders to influence health systems, and to develop health care policy that includes an awareness of health disparities through the application of culturally proficient care. The DNP programs are in their initial stages of implementation and have had a tremendous response from practicing nurses. Just as in a nurse practitioner program, there are many areas in which to specialize, from family to mental health to education. Read more about this new opportunity on the AACN site (http://www.aacn.org).

CONCLUSION

For many, returning to school is a big decision, a life-changing choice, and a personal goal. Rozy is most articulate about her decision:

I am also guided by the spiritual path I walk, and, frankly, I feel led to attend graduate school. At times, this knowledge is all that gets me through a rough week of work at the hospital, clinicals, classes, cases, family needs, and fatigue. It also helps to have a cheering section of my husband, daughter, brothers, my father, and friends. It helps that they believe in the awesome field of nursing as well as in me. One of my brothers told me recently how much he enjoyed telling others, "My sister is a nurse." I told him that coincidentally, I love saying, "I am a nurse."

Education will empower you to be a knowledgeable and skilled nurse. Years ago, at one of our Academic Rounds presentations, in standing room only full of undergraduate, Master's, and doctoral students, I had the privilege of introducing one of our great leaders, the esteemed Virginia Henderson, nurse theorist and pioneer, who at the time, was 90 years old. A member of the audience raised her hand and asked what level of education Professor Henderson thought a nurse should have. Without skipping a beat, Professor Henderson responded with, "The nurse should have the highest level of education attainable so she will be more able to care for the widest breadth of patients." Education offers you opportunities and as Professor Henderson acknowledged, it benefits the patient and the public we serve.

END-OF-CHAPTER EXERCISE

Now that you have been a staff nurse for a while, where do you see yourself in 5 years?

- Are you at the bedside? Consider the CNL degree (http://www.aacn.nche.edu/CNL/).

- Do you see yourself functioning as a nurse practitioner (http://www.aacn.nche.edu/DNP/index.htm)?
- There are many specialties for a nurse practitioner (http://www.aanp.org/default.asp).
- Certified Nurse-Midwives (CNMs) (http://www.acnm.org/).
- Certified Registered Nurse Anesthetists (CRNAs) (http://www.aana.com/).
- Are you considering teaching? There are the PhD and the DNP options. (http://www.preparing-faculty.org).
- What about a nurse scientist? (http://www.aacn.nche.edu/Publications/positions/qualityindicators.htm).
- Look at the reference list in this chapter. You may want to read a few of the articles.
- Check out the fast track from BS to PhD (http://www.aacn.nche.edu/Publications/AcceleratedPrograms.htm).

Consider all the options. One option will fit your goals.

References

American Association of Colleges of Nursing. (1996). *The essentials of master's education for advanced practice nursing.* Washington, DC: American Association of Colleges of Nursing.

Berkenkotter, C., Huckin, T., & Ackerman, J. (1999). Conventions, conversations and the writer: Case study of a student in a rhetoric PhD program. *Research in the Teaching of English, 22*(1), 9–44.

Chandler, G. (1991). Creating an empowered environment. *Nursing Management, 22*(8), 20–23.

Chandler, G. (1999). A creative writing intervention to enhance self esteem and self efficacy in adolescents. *Journal of Child and Adolescent Psychiatric Nursing, 12*(2), 70–78.

Lamott, A. (1995). *Bird by bird.* New York: Anchor Books.

McIntosh, P. (1985). *Feeling like a fraud: Work in progress.* Wellesley, MA: Wellesley Centers for Women.

Schneider, P. (2003). *Writing alone and with others.* New York: Oxford University Press.

A Sample
of Assignments
Required in
an Introductory
Nursing Course

Identify a historical figure, their credentials, contributions, time/era, and describe whether today if what they contributed is pertinent or not. Reflect on your learning.

Research a health topic of interest, such as binge drinking or eating disorders; identify a study and the salient points.

Find out what certification means and interview a nurse certified in a specialty area.

Review the Healthy People 2010 document, choose a topic, and research what is known about the topic.

Read a legal and ethical case study, apply terminology, Code of Ethics, and your opinion.

Conduct a self cultural diversity or a sociocultural evaluation. Write a reflective response.

Research spirituality in health care. Read nurse narratives and *Chicken Soup for the Nurse's Soul.*

Study palliative care, the collaboration between patient and hospice, and the teamwork approach; research case studies.

NCLEX Preparation Resources

Question Resources

NCLEX Review 3500 CD-ROM (2005). Philadelphia: Lippincott Williams & Wilkins.

Silvestri, L. (2006). *Saunders Question and Answer Review for NCLEX-RN* (3rd ed.). St. Louis, MO: Saunders Elsevier.

Saxton, D., Nugent, P., Pelikan, P., & Green, J. (2005). *Mosby's review questions for the NCLEX-RN ® examination* (5th ed.). St. Louis, MO: Elsevier, Inc.

NCLEX-RN 250 new format questions. (2007). Philadelphia: Lippincott Williams and Wilkins.

Pharmacology Resources

Hogan, M. (Ed.). (2005). *Pharmacology: Reviews and rationales.* Upper Saddle River, NJ: Prentice Hall.

Waide, L., & Roland, B. (2001). *Pharmacology made easy for the NCLEX-RN.* Chicago Review Press.

Zerwekh, J., Claborn, J., & Gagliano. (2005). *Mosby's Pharmacology NoteCards: Visual, mnemonic and memory aids for nurses.* St. Louis, MO: Mosby Elsevier.

Test-Taking Strategies Resources

Kaplan "NCLEX-RN: Strategies for the Registered Nursing licensing exam" 2007 edition

Silvestri, L. (2005). *Saunders strategies for success for the NCLEX-RN Examination* (1st ed.). St. Louis, MO: Saunders Elsevier.

Kaplan. (2005). *NCLEX-RN Exam 2005–2006.* New York: Kaplan.

Hoefler, P. (2004). *Successful problem solving and test-taking for beginning nursing students.* Meds Incorporated.

Nugent, P. M., & Vitale, B. A. (2004). *Test success: Test taking techniques for beginning nursing students* (4th ed.). Philadelphia: F. A. Davis.

Contact Information for NCLEX-RN Preparation Review Courses Online or In-Person

Linda Silvestri 800 598–6730; http://www.us.elsevierhealth.com/

Barbara Murphy 978–486–3137

Kaplan Review Course 1–800–533–8850

NCLEX-RN Practice Computer Adaptive Test Simulation

Mosby's Computer Adaptive Test (CAT) For NCLEX-RN Examination On Line. (2004). 2nd ed. http://www.us.elsevierhealth.com/product.jsp?isbn=0323032524.

ATI testing—http://www.atitesting.co

Web Sites with Information for Students Attending an AD (Two-Year) Degree or a BS (Four-Year) Degree Program

Practice Area	Description	Web Site
Medical/Surgical Nursing	General nursing	American Academy of Medical-Surgical Nurses http://www.medsurgnurse.org
Labor and Delivery	Families and babies	http://www.awhonn.org
Postpartum	Families and babies	http://www.awhonn.org
Neo-Natal Intensive Care	Families and babies	http://www.nann.org http://www.awhonn.org

(Continued)

Pediatrics	Working with newborn to 18-year-olds on a general pediatric unit or a specialty unit such as respiratory, neurology, PICU, or pediatric rehabilitation.	http://www. pedsnurses.org/ http://www. pediatricnursing.com http://www.napnap
Perioperative	Operating room	http://www.aorn.org/
Emergency Nurse	ER education, certification, and research	http://www.ena.org/
Orthopedic	Education certification and research	http://www.orthonurse.org/
Oncology	Cancer nursing	http://www.ons.org/
Critical Care	Intensive care nursing	http://www.aacn.org
Outpatient clinic		
Gerontology	Caring for the older adult	http://www.ngna.org/
Rehabilitation	Caring for patients in rehabilitation settings	http://www. rehab-nurse.org
Long-Term Care		http://www.ngna.org/
Hospice	Palliative care nursing	http://www.hpna.org/
Home Care	Visiting nurses	http://www.vnaa.org
Mental Health	Psychiatric nursing	http://www.apna.org

Index

A

AACN (*see* American Association of Colleges of Nursing)
Academic writing, 188
Acceptance stage, 107–108
AD in nursing (*see* Associate's degree in nursing)
AD to BS program, 42–45, 51
Adjustment, stages of, 105–108
Administering inverventions, 24
Administration, dealing with, 75
Admission processes, 31
Admissions Committee, 81, 98
Advanced Practice Core Curriculum, 174
Advanced-beginner stage, 142–143
Advocacy, patient, 13–14, 76–77
Affordability, of nursing school, 94–98
  federal/state assistance, 96, 97
  local assistance, 96, 97
Agency for Healthcare Research and Quality (AHRQ), 187
American Association for Nurses, 58
American Association of Colleges of Nursing (AACN), 49–50, 58, 173
American Journal of Nursing, 50
American Nurses Association, 147
American Nurses' Credentialing Center (ANCC), 147
American Psychological Association (APA):
  manual from, 187–188
  writing format of, 119
Amherst Writers and Artists' method, 189–190
Anatomy, 30
ANCC (American Nurses' Credentialing Center), 147
APA (*see* American Psychological Association)
Application/applying to nursing school, 81–103
  and affordability, 94–98
  and alternatives to nursing school, 102
  and campus visit, 98
  checklist for, 95
  Common Undergraduate Application for, 62
  essay for, 82–92
  and interview, 98–102
  letters of recommendation for, 92–94
  planning for, 72
  and student status, 61
  themes for developing successful, 60
  website resources for, 73
Arrien, Angeles, 128
Asking questions, 75, 126, 127
Assertiveness, 76–77
Assessment:
  of patient, 2, 5
  self- (*see* Self-assessment (for nursing school))
Assignments:
  back-planning of, 118–122
  and nursing-school success, 122–123
  and organization, 117–118
  sample, 195
Assimilation stage, 108
Assistance, financial, 94–98
Associate's degree (AD) in nursing:
  BS after, 42–45, 51
  description, 41, 51
  web sites for, 199–200
Asynchronous learning, 43
Auxiliary nurses, use of, 142

B

Baccalaureate degree in another field, 173
Bachelor of Science (BS) degree in nursing, 45–49
  after Associate's Degree, 42–45
  description, 45, 51

Bachelor of Science (BS) degree in
     nursing (*Cont.*):
  path leading to, 45–48
  reality of, 48–49
  as second degree, 49–50
  web sites for, 199–200
Back-planning, 118–122
Balance:
  of career and life, 38–40
  of school and family, 134–135
Beck, Cheryl, 36
Benner, P., 20–21
Benner, Patricia, 12, 140
Bereavement (example), 3–4
"Bird-by-bird" analogy, 122–123
Birth control, 7
Bodily-kinesthetic intelligence, 65
Books, 115, 116
Breaks, taking, 130–131
Bridges, W., 139
BS in nursing (*see* Bachelor of Science
     degree in nursing)
Burnout, 38–40

C
Cameron, Julia, 88, 132
Campus visit, 86, 98
Career, nursing (*see* Nursing career)
Career fairs, 148
Career services, 148
Caring:
  for patients, 34–35
  for self, 39, 129–134
Center for Disease Control (CDC),
     187
Center for Nurse Advocacy, 148
Certified Nursing Assistant (CNA),
     67, 110, 112, 114
CEUs (continuing education units),
     162
Changing conditions, effective
     management of rapidly, 22–24
Chemistry, 30
CINAHL, 174
Clinical Institute Withdrawal
     Assessment for Alcohol (CIWA), 25

Clinical Nurse Leader (CNL),
     50, 175
Clinical Nurse Specialist (CNS), 175
Clinical setting(s):
  and class work, 46–48
  early exposure to, 30–31
  experience with, 109–116
  local vs. international, 188
  preparation for, 124–125
  principles of harmony/balance for,
     128
  research in, 31
Clustering, 86
CNA (*see* Certified Nursing Assistant)
CNL (*see* Clinical Nurse Leader)
CNS (Clinical Nurse Specialist), 175
Coaching, 17–20
Collaboration, 16
Comfort, providing, 3–4
Common Undergraduate Application,
     62
Communication, 11–12, 14
Community service, 66–67
Competent-nurse stage, 143
Computer adaptive test simulation, 198
Conferences, nursing, 174–175
Confidence, 112
Connections, 133–134
Continuing education units (CEUs),
     162
Coursework:
  and application process, 63–64
  general education, 45
  general vs. specialty, 46–47
  prenursing requirements, 30
Cover letters, 150, 152–153
Creativity, on essay, 86–89
  free-writing, 87–89
  mind maps, 86–87
Crimean War, 7
Curiosity, 75–76
Curriculum, graduate, 174

D
Defibrillators, 23
Delegation, 114

Diagnostic function, 20–22
Dignity, 17
Diploma programs, 51
Direct Loan, 97
Direct-entry graduate degree
    in nursing, 50, 52
DNP (*see* Doctorate of Nursing
    Practice)
Doctoral degree (PhD) in nursing,
    50, 52, 190–192
Doctorate of Nursing Practice (DNP),
    50, 52, 192–193
Drafting, 90
Dressing (for interviews), 101–102,
    156
Duckling model, 125

E
Editing, 91
Edmondson, A., 161
Education:
    nursing, 106, 176–177
    as résumé listing, 149
Elbow, P., 87–88
Email address, 149
Emotional concerns, 4
Empowerment, 188–189
Environment, nursing, 166–167
Essays, application, 82–92
    and creativity, 86–89
    following directions for, 82–83
    and school's web site, 84–86
    and stages of writing, 89–92
"Essentials of Master's Education"
    (AACN), 173–174
Excitement, 35
Exercise, physical, 131
Exhaustion, 39
Experience:
    journals/books about nurses', 115
    and nursing-school success, 109–116
    as résumé listing, 149
    and transition to nursing, 164–166
Expert nurses, 39, 133
Expert-nurse stage, 143
Extracurricular activities, 66–67

F
Facebook pages, 153
FAFSA (Free Application for Federal
    Student Aid), 96
Family, of patient:
    comforting, 3–4
    liaison for, 16–17
    teaching, 19
Family life, 134–135
Family Nurse Practitioner, 176
Family support, 134, 136
Fast track programs, 173
Federal assistance, 96, 97
Federal Need Analysis Methodology, 95
Federal Work Study (FWS) program, 97
Final draft, 91–92
Financial assistance, 94–98
Flexible schedule, 37–38, 40
Floating (among nursing units), 38
Foundation of the National Student
    Nurses Association, 96
Fraud, feeling like a, 184
Free Application for Federal Student
    Aid (FAFSA), 96
Free-writing, 87–89
Friendships, 32, 131–132
Fundamentals of nursing (courses),
    46–47
FWS (Federal Work Study) program,
    97

G
Gardner, Howard, 64
GPA (*see* Grade point average)
Grade point average (GPA), 31, 32,
    62–63
Graduate Core Curriculum, 174
Graduate degree in nursing, 50
Graduate school, 171–193
    curriculum of, 174
    decision making about, 174–175
    description of, 185–190
    direct entry to, 50
    doctoral programs in, 190–192
    goal of, 173–174
    imposter syndrome, 182–185

Graduate school (*Cont.*):
  informational sessions for, 180
  network support for, 181–182
  rationale for entering, 172–173
  resources for, 180–181
  self-assessment for, 178–180
  specialty areas in, 175–177
GRE review course, 183
Griffin, Martha, 166

H
Hayes, Eileen, 163
Health care issues, 106
Healthy People 2010, 106
Helping role, 13–17
Henderson, Virginia, 7
Hierarchies, 184, 185
Honeymoon stage, 105–106
Humor, 165

I
Imposter syndrome, 42, 182–185
Informational sessions (for nursing
  programs), 180
Institute of Medicine (IOM), 72, 106
Intelligences, 64–65
Interactive video programs, 43
Internal critic, 183–184
Internship, 48
Interpersonal intelligence, 65
Interview(s):
  dressing for, 101–102, 156
  for jobs, 153–156
  for nursing school, 98–102
  practice for, 155
  thank-you note following, 156
  work environment, 167
Intrapersonal intelligence, 65
Introductory course in nursing, 46, 195
Inverventions, administering/
  monitoring, 24
IOM (*see* Institute of Medicine)

J
Job search, 147–156
  and career services, 148
  and cover letters, 150, 152–153

and interviews, 153–156
  résumés for, 148–152

K
Knowledge workers, 2

L
Lamott, Anne, 122, 183
Leadership, 68–72
Letters of recommendation,
  92–94, 111
Liaison for family, 16–17
Licensed Practical Nurse (LPN), 41
Licensed Vocational Nurse (LVN), 41
Licensing exam:
  for AD, 41
  for LPN/LVN, 41
  NCLEX (*see* National Counsel
    Licensing Exam)
Linguistic intelligence, 64
Listening, 8–10, 16
Loans, 94–97
Logical-mathematical intelligence, 64
LPN (Licensed Practical Nurse), 41
LVN (Licensed Vocational Nurse), 41

M
Magnet status, 147–148
Mandatory overtime policies, 38
Master's degree in nursing, 50, 52
McIntosh, Peg, 184
Mentors:
  faculty, 139
  finding, 163–164
  in nursing school, 137
Microbiology, 30
Mind maps, 86–87
Mobility, 38, 40
Musical intelligence, 65

N
National Counsel Licensing Exam
  (NCLEX), 143–146
  preparation for, 144–146
  preparation resources for, 197–198
  review course for, 144
National Institutes of Health (NIH), 187

Naturalist intelligence, 65
NCLEX (*see* National Counsel Licensing Exam)
Neighborhood health programs, 7
Networks, support (*see* Support networks)
New grad groups, 160–161
Nightingale, Florence, 7, 76, 137
NIH (National Institutes of Health), 187
Nontraditional students, 135–137
Novice-nurse stage, 141–142
NP (*see* Nurse Practitioner)
Nurse managers, 161
Nurse Practitioner (NP), 175, 176
Nurse preceptors, 48, 162
Nurses:
  critical role of, 55–57
  function of, 7
Nursing, 1–27
  administering-/monitoring-inverventions role of, 24
  bereavement example, 3–4
  as career, 37–40
  caring aspect of, 34–35
  and communication, 11–12
  definition of, 9
  diagnostic/monitoring role of, 20–22
  excitement of, 35
  familiarity with, 33–34
  helping role of, 13–17
  history of, 6–7
  impact of, 35–36
  organizational role of, 25–26
  pediatrics example, 1–2
  quality-/safety-management role of, 24–25
  and rapidly changing conditions, effective management of, 22–24
  rehabilitation example, 8–11
  roles of, 12–13
  school nurse example, 4–5
  as science, 36–37
  teaching-coaching role of, 17–20
Nursing career, 37–40
  and burnout, 38–40
  and flexible schedule, 37–38, 40
  and mobility, 38, 40

Nursing conferences, 174–175
Nursing education, 106, 176–177
Nursing journals, 115
Nursing program(s), 40–52
  AD, 41
  AD to BS, 42–45
  BS, 45–49
  direct-entry graduate, 50
  LPN, 41
  online, 43–45
  options in, 51–52
  second-degree, 49–50
Nursing Reinvestment Act, 96
Nursing school, 29–32
  admission to, 31
  clinical aspect of, 30–31
  courses required in, 30
  demanding schedule of, 29
  and GPA, 31, 32
  research aspect of, 31
  social life, 32
Nursing Student loan, 97
Nursing-school success, 105–138
  assignments, 122–123
  back-planning, 118–122
  experience, 109–116
  family life, 134–135
  mentors for, 137
  for nontraditional students, 135–137
  and organization, 116–118
  and stages of adjustment, 105–108
  and stress management, 129–134
  and time management, 123–129

O

Offensive behavior, 166
Online programs:
  for NCLEX preparation, 198
  for nursing, 43–45
  for RN mobility, 173
Organization tools, 117
Organizational role, 25–26
Organizational skills, 46, 61–72
  and extracurricular activities/community service, 66–67
  and GPA/coursework, 62–66

Organizational skills (*Cont.*):
  and leadership, 68–72
  and nursing-school success, 116–118
Orientation, job, 159–161
Overtime policies, 38

P
Pain management, 13–14
Parent Loan for Undergraduate
  Students (PLUS), 97
Pathophysiology, 30
Patient advocates, 13–14, 76–77
Patient safety, 106, 167
Pediatrics (example), 1–2
Peer networking, 126–127, 136–137,
  160–161
Peer pressure, 32
Pell grant, 97
Pellico, Linda, 50
Per diem staff, 142
Perkins loan, 97
Personal inventory, 58–61
PhD in nursing (*see* Doctoral degree
  in nursing)
Physical concerns, 4
Physical exercise, 131
PLUS (Parent Loan for Undergraduate
  Students), 97
Prenursing programs, 31
Prewriting, 89
Procedures, 141
Proficient-nurse stage, 143
Proofreading, 91
PubMed, 174

Q
Quality management, 24–25

R
Rapidly changing conditions, effective
  management of, 22–24
Reflection, 65
Registered nurses (RNs):
  AD program for, 41
  AD-to-BS program for, 42–45
  from LPNs, 41
Rehabilitation (example), 8–11

Rejection stage, 107
Relationships:
  building, 73–75
  and nursing-school success,
    133–134
Research, in nursing school, 31
Research assistants, 97
Resources, for graduate school,
  180–181
Résumés, 148–152
  computer vs. "going-out-the-door,"
    149
  and letters of recommendation, 93
  sample, 151–152
  workshops for writing, 148
Review courses, 144
Revising, 90–91
RN Mobility program, 173
RNs (*see* Registered nurses)
Roberts, Sue, 166
Role development, 140–141
Rules, 141

S
Safety, patient, 106, 167
Safety management, 24–25
Sample assignments, 195
Sanger, Margaret, 7
SAR (Student Aid report), 96
Schneider, Pat, 189
Scholarships, 94–97, 116
School nurse (example), 4–5
Science, nursing as, 36–37
Second degree programs in nursing,
  49–50, 52
Self-assessment (for nursing school),
  55–78
  assertiveness, 76–77
  curiosity, 75–76
  extracurricular activities/community
    service, 66–67
  GPA/coursework, 62–66
  for graduate school, 178–180
  leadership, 68–73
  organization, 61–73
  personal inventory, 58–61
  relationship building, 73–75

Senior staff availability, 142
SEOG (Supplemental Educational
   Opportunity Grant), 97
September 11, 2001 terrorist attacks,
   186
Shock stage, 106–107
"Sim Man," 123
SNAP (student nursing assistant
   program), 94
Social life, 32
Social support, 157–158
Spatial intelligence, 65
Specialty classes, 47
Specialty organizations, 174, 181
Staff development, 162
Staffing, 142
State assistance, 96, 97
Stress management, 129–134
   with breaks, 130–131
   with diversion, 133
   and NCLEX, 145
   with physical exercise, 131
   with relationships, 133–134
   with venting, 131–132
Student Aid report (SAR), 96
Student nursing assistant program
   (SNAP), 94
Study habits, 46, 145
Supplemental Educational Opportunity
   Grant (SEOG), 97
Support networks:
   in clinical settings, 126–127
   for graduate school, 181–182
   in life, 189–190
   mentors in, 163–164
   for new nurses, 157–164
   nurse manager in, 161
   nurse preceptor in, 162
   orientation, 159–161
Surveillance, 167

T
Teachable moments, 18–20
Teaching, 17–20
Textbooks, 116
Thank-you notes, 156

Time management:
   importance of, 46
   and nursing-school success, 123–129
Touch, 14
Transition, student–nurse, 139–168
   advanced-beginner stage of,
      142–143
   competent/proficient/expert stages
      of, 143
   components of successful, 140
   and experience/environment, 164–168
   and job search (*see* Job search)
   and NCLEX, 143–146
   novice-nurse stage of, 141–142
   and stages of role development,
      140–141
   and support networks, 157–164
Travel nurses, 38
Tucker, A., 161
Tuition reimbursement programs, 94

U
U.S. Department of Education, 96
University of Washington, 111

V
Venting, 131–132
Voice, developing and using your, 167
Volunteering, 74, 110, 111

W
Wald, Lillian, 7
web sites:
   hospital, 73
   and image of school, 84–86
   for nurses, 199–200
Work load expectations, 142
Work study program, 97
Work-to-pay-back loan programs, 97
Writer's block, 89
Writing:
   academic, 188
   APA format for, 119
   free-, 87–89
   stages of, 89–92
   as stress reliever, 132